Amazon

"This book is fantastic! Real, genuine and bare-naked honest. If you are looking for quick fixes, gimmicks and a complicated diet plan, don't buy this book. If you are looking for straightforward open inspiration, this is it! Refreshing, in this instant gratification world, someone finally motivates with true success and no self-promotion. Bryan's success and straight talk speaks for itself. Bryan gets by with being painfully honest because one, he lives what he preaches, and two, his goal is to truly inspire others, without his ego in the way. Most true heroes never need to boast or brag. Their life alone is a testimony of their tenacity, integrity and courage. You will not regret buying this book."

"I found Bryan's story to be very inspirational. He's a guy that's speaking from his heart and not from a Ph.D, so don't expect to get a lot of science in this book. Bryan is just telling us what worked for him personally. Follow Bryan's advice and get professional coaching and guidance before you make any drastic changes to your diet and exercise--but then follow through on it. Bryan's story will motivate you to get started on your journey to a healthier and happier life. He doesn't pull any punches when he talks about the fast food and weight loss gimmick industries--he hates them!"

"Even if you don't have a weight issue, perhaps your neighbor, co-worker, or another family member does. Read this book. Some of Bryan's common sense can be applied to other lifestyle changes you might need to make. I found this to be an enjoyable, easy read. Bryan pulls no punches by describing what worked for him. Will it work for you? Only you can judge and only if you read this book."

*Courtesy of Amazon.com, Inc. or its affiliates. All rights reserved.

IMPOSSIBLE

How I Lost Nearly 400 Pounds Without Surgery

By Bryan Ganey

Copyright 2013, By Bryan Ganey. All rights reserved. No part of this book may be used or reproduced in any manner whatsoever without the written permission of the author.

Cover photos courtesy of Erin Honious, taken at Isle of Palms, South Carolina.

CONTENTS

What This Book Is And What It Isn't - 11
Why Read This Book – 13
My Wake-Up Call - 18
Coming Home: Now What? Getting Started - 24
Changing Your Mindset – You Are The 5% - 29
The Mental Block - 34
Breaking All The Rules: Weight Loss Myths - 40
Time To Change Your Lifestyle - 48
The 4 Steps To Successful, Long-Term Weight Management - 56
The Disappointment Machine - 65
Just Say No To The Force Feeders - 70
Food Is Not A Reward - 73
Stay Humble, My Friends - 75
Portion Distortion - 79
Settling And Dying Happy - 81
Priorities - 83
Why Not Just Stop? - 86
Rage Against The Weight Loss Machine - 88
Restaurant Addiction – 94
Make Your Bucket List - 100
The Wrong Idea About Eating - 103
What Do I Eat? Yes, There Are Bad Foods - 105
When You Struggle (And You Will) - 109
Workout Music - 112
The Great Clothes Line - 114
Failure Is A Gift - 116
One More Time: There Is No Secret   118
Why Not Have Weight Loss Surgery? - 121
The 7 Habits Of Healthy People - 123
Walking Is The Exercise Gateway Drug - 126
When You Get To The End, You Won! - 128
Fat Shaming? Are You Kidding Me? - 130
An Open Letter To The Weight Loss Industry - 133
Pictures - 135

ABOUT THE AUTHOR

Bryan Ganey was born and raised in Dayton, Ohio. After 32 years, he relocated to his adopted hometown of Charleston, South Carolina. Bryan has spent the last 3 years changing his life, losing nearly 400 pounds and has started a career as an author and motivational speaker.

http://www.bryanganey.com

e-mail: ganeybooks@gmail.com

Twitter: @bganey

Facebook: http://www.facebook.com/ganeyinc

YouTube Channel: http://www.youtube.com/bganey

ACKNOWLEDGEMENTS

First and foremost, I would like to thank my family, without whom I wouldn't be here (and would have died 3 years ago had they not taken me to the hospital.) Their unconditional love and support has meant the world to me. I would like to thank all of my close friends who have supported me throughout this journey. You know who you are.

I would like to thank all of the doctors and nurses who have treated me. I could name names, but I would forget somebody, so I will just leave it at that. I would also like to thank my health and wellness coaches, who have always been there to push me to my absolute limit.

And last but not least, I would like to thank all of the readers of my blog, followers on Facebook, Twitter and everyone who has e-mailed me over the years with their stories of struggle. I have made so many new friends all over the world. If I listed them all, it would take up 50 pages and would be boring to read, so I won't.

Now on with the book.

DISCLAIMER

The information contained in this book is for informational purposes only. Bryan Ganey is not a qualified health professional, just a regular guy that lost a bunch of weight on his own.

Please seek medical advice from a doctor before beginning any weight loss program. Please seek nutritional advice from a registered dietitian prior to beginning any weight loss program. Please consult a medical doctor before beginning any exercise program. Please also consult a certified personal trainer before beginning any exercise program.

The decision to have or not have weight loss surgery is a decision that you should make after consulting with your doctor and doing your own appropriate research. Do not make that decision based on anything you read in this book.

Do not follow anything you read in this book without discussing it with your doctor first. By reading this book, you are agreeing that you will take your health seriously and only proceed with a lifestyle change after receiving sound medical advice from a qualified health professional.

This book, anything contained in it and anything said or written by Bryan Ganey should not be considered qualified, professional medical advice nor should any of it be followed without consulting a physician first.

ABOUT THE TITLE

Three years ago, I saw a new doctor for the first time. Like every doctor before him, he immediately began pushing weight loss surgery.

As I sat there talking to him, I weighed 577 pounds and was covered in bruises from having blood thinners pumped into me for 6 days in the hospital. I dared to ask the question:

"What if I lost the weight on my own?"

This doctor was quick to shoot it down: "It would be **impossible**."

The word hit me like a ton of bricks. Impossible? I started to think: time travel is impossible. Escaping death and taxes is impossible.

But losing weight is not impossible, no matter how big the number. It may be difficult, it may take a long time, there may be setbacks, I may not always like what I have to do.

But it is **not** impossible.

I walked out of that office and never looked back. I never saw that doctor again, nor will I. I was determined this time would be different. I was going to do it my way. And I was going to make it last.

As for that doctor? No, I have no interest in going back and seeing him and saying "I told you so." I did this for myself, not for anyone else or any other reason.

THE NO 'O-WORD' PLEDGE

I, Bryan Ganey, hereby do pledge to you that I will never use the "O-Word" anywhere in this book.

What is the "O-word?" You know the word. I will use it once so you know what I am talking about: obese. It is the word that society and the media use to stereotype the overweight. It has been used as a label with such frequency and with such condescension that I now hate it.

In my opinion, it is an absolute irrefutable fact that the last acceptable form of discrimination in our society is the mistreatment of the overweight. It isn't right, but a large portion of society sees big people as less than a human being, if they see them at all. I've experienced this first hand. You are due the same respect any other person is so don't tolerate the jokes, the put-downs or the comments.

You are a person with as much to offer as anyone else. I will not devalue you by labeling you with the "O-Word."

Since this is my book, you will never read that word in this book again.

WHAT THIS BOOK IS AND WHAT IT ISN'T

This is not a diet book. If you're looking for somebody to lose the weight for you, they don't exist. If you're looking for the quick fix, this isn't it. There is no quick fix, so stop looking for one.

Throughout this book, I will repeat myself a lot. Why? Because what I am advocating is simple common sense. I am going to say it over and over again.

But if you're like I was….you've had enough of the lies, the scams, the rip-offs, the gimmicks…then this is the book for you. I will give it to you straight because that is the way I want it given to me.

The reason you read a book like this is not to find out how to lose weight. You know how to do that. Eat less and exercise more. That's all. The reason you buy a book like this is to see what you can learn about the approach and the mindset. You want my success so you want to see what you can learn from me.

Unlike almost everyone else, I will not lie to you. No more lies. It ends now and it ends here. No more. Say it out loud while you pound your fist on the table: NO MORE!

And finally, like the disclaimer at the beginning of the book says, I am not a professional. I am a regular guy. As a society, we need to stop taking medical advice from people we see on TV and read on the Internet. After you read my book, go see your doctor. Talk about losing weight the healthy way. Come up with a plan of action. Get a referral for a good registered dietitian. Learn about healthy, well-balanced meals.

Remember: the harder it is, the better. The more you struggle, the better. You want it to be difficult because that is how you earn your success. That is how you make it last.

You will see a lot of lists in this book. Why? I make lists. Lots of lists. To-do lists. Grocery lists. My daily food journal is a list. Lists help me organize my life. So almost every chapter has a list.

One last note: I have to apologize to my English teacher at Stivers School for the Arts in Dayton, Ohio. I am an unconventional writer. I will start sentences with "And." I will use too many commas. I use the word "you" a lot. Some sentences will be fragments. I did the best I could, Mrs. Schaetzle.

WHY READ THIS BOOK?

There are thousands of diet books. All of them have experienced varying degrees of popularity and they will all make you lose weight.

So why am I different?

Here's why my way will work. It is designed to last. I am not going to sit here and insult your intelligence and tell you that it is easy once you get started. It isn't. All diets will give you that temporary euphoria of winning. It all ends the same way...6 or 9 months or a year of success...only to fall back down to the bottom of a deep, dark hole of depression and despair when you can't keep up the diet. The old habits return and you're back at square one. Why even bother?

There are 10,000 ways to lose weight, but only one way to keep it off. Enter my plan.

First of all, I have lived it. I have lost nearly 400 pounds on my own, with no pills, no surgery, no diets and no gimmicks. Granted, what works for one person might not work for another. But I will tell you what doesn't work: temporary fad diets with a proven record of failure.

Second, I am going to tell you the common sense you already know. I am going to tell you to see a doctor before you try to lose weight. I am going to say it over and over. I am going to tell you to visit a registered dietitian before you begin. Where my expertise comes in is the application of common-sense weight loss principles.

I will tell you how to avoid all of the common pitfalls and traps that people fall into, because I have already fallen into them. I have already done the work for you. By purchasing this book and reading it, you get to experience my success and my failures, without having to live through it yourself.

So fasten your seatbelt (even if you have to get a seatbelt extender.) It's going to be a fun ride.

You can do this. Any fool can lose weight. But to keep it off for the rest of your life…that's the challenge.

The one question I have consistently been asked again and again over the last 3 years is this:

"Where does the motivation come from and how do I get it?"

I'll tell you where it comes from. It comes from being absolutely, 100%, without question, fed up with my situation. It comes from being sick and tired of being sick and tired.

It comes from shaking your fist at the sky and screaming..."I AM NOT GOING TO TAKE ANY MORE!!!"

I have a fire...a RAGE that burns inside me on a daily basis. It is an anger that drives me. If you have a big lifestyle change you want to undergo, I recommend getting ANGRY and FIRED UP. You're going to need it.

Three years ago I was hospitalized due to complications from being overweight. For 6 days I laid there in my own filth because I was unable to shower and I remember saying over and over: NO MORE. There will be NO MORE of this. I remember making a list of all the things there would be NO MORE of:

-There would be no more of me relying on other people to help me get out of bed, to help me get around.
-There will be no more of me being so heavy and immobile that another person has to help me go to the bathroom.
-There will be no more of me needing life-saving tests done at the hospital and being told I am "too big for the machine."
-There will be no more being so heavy, the biggest clothes in the Big and Tall store are too small.
-There will be no more being too big to drive a car.
-There will be no more riding in the elevator and being unable to take the stairs.
-There will be no more making my family and friends worry about me dropping dead at any time.
-There will be no more prescriptions.
-There will be no more sympathy from people you don't want it from.
-There will be no more pity.
-There will be no more people telling me that I can't do it myself.
-There will be no more people recommending weight loss surgery to me.
-There will be no more hospitals.
-There will be no more blood clots.
-There will be no more of me eating myself to death.

No more. And here we are 3 years later. That's where my motivation comes from.

Simply losing weight should never be the focus. As a matter of fact, it's a counterproductive way to think. Being overweight is a symptom of an unhealthy lifestyle, it is not the cause of it.
Before you start thinking about losing weight and trying to add years

to your life and life to your years, you have to be in the proper frame of mind. You need to think about how you can make your lifestyle change permanent. If all you're going to do is temporarily change what you do in order to lose 50 pounds for a wedding and then put it all back on, you may as well not bother.

No, what you want is a total lifestyle change. Nothing less will do. That is the best chance you have at getting healthier, losing weight, keeping it off and staying out of the doctor's office. So what are the steps that go into this? First, you have to analyze your own behavior. You know yourself better than anyone else, right?

Identify what your demons are and stay away from them....forever. For me, one of my biggest demons is restaurants. When I am being served food in a restaurant, I cannot control myself. It is very much like an alcoholic in a bar. So I stay far, far away. For you, it might be something simple like mindless eating. Whatever it is, identify it and don't do it!

For a successful lifestyle change, you need two things: proper nutrition and exercise. This sounds like an impossible, huge task, but it's not. I have had great success eating 3 large meals per day and 3 snacks, totaling about 2,800-3,000 calories: fruits, vegetables, lean meats, beans, rice, low fat dairy and whole grains. And lots and lots of water. Keep a food journal. Nothing goes into the hole in your head called your mouth without writing it down. Pack your lunch every day and eat what you pack. No restaurants. Never let someone else decide what you're going to eat and how much you're going to eat. You're not a dog...you don't just eat what's in the bowl because your master put it there.

Now for the exercise. Talk to your doctor about what he or she recommends and start where you are. My first exercises were pushing a grocery cart around the store and walking to my mailbox at the end of my driveway. It was all I could do. But the key to my success is consistency. Exercise should NOT be painful. ('No pain, no gain' is a lie.) But what exercise should do is elevate your heart rate and build your strength and stamina. Start out slowly. The biggest mistake people make is going all-out and burning themselves out before they even get started. Work out 3 times a week, with a day off in between and off on the weekend. You must allow your body time to recover. Walking is the best exercise to start with. Don't even bother with a gym membership at first. Walk 5, 10, 15 and eventually 30 minutes a day, 3 times a week. Once you have that conquered, increase the time. Then look for hills to climb, and so on.

Remember: slow and steady wins the race. You are changing your life. Oh, and one final tip: stay off the scale. Weigh once at the start, then about once a month. Being obsessed by the scale and weighing constantly will only fuel your disappointment.

You can do it. You know you can and so do I. Take your life back. Take it back starting right now.

MY WAKE-UP CALL

On June 20, 2010, my life changed forever.

I was 37 years old. I had been overweight my entire life and had long given up doing anything about it. Like many people, I tried the diets and they all failed me. None of it worked because none of it was ever going to work. Sure, I lost weight, but I always gained it all back plus more.

So I gave up. I just figured I would be heavy the rest of my life, however long that lasted. I got bigger and bigger. 360 pounds became 400 pounds turned into 450 pounds and then one day I hit 500 pounds. There seemed to be no limit to how much weight I would gain and I seemed powerless to stop it.

Food was my drug and I was addicted. I could not stop eating. While others would be out socializing and enjoying life, I would be sitting in my apartment by myself binge eating pizza, ice cream, fast food and every junk food item imaginable.

As I started to get older, the consequences of my food abuse began to show more and more. I developed high blood pressure. Then came an irregular heartbeat, apparently a result of my 12-can-a-day diet soda habit. I developed sleep apnea. I was on multiple medications for conditions that were not normal for an otherwise healthy adult in their 30's. Then my mobility started becoming restricted. I started having difficulty getting out of bed in the morning. If I fell, it took 2 strong people to help me up. I couldn't put my shoes on by myself anymore. I couldn't buy clothes from anywhere anymore. Everything in the big and tall store was too small. All of my clothes had to be specially tailored to fit me. The size 7X underwear that I mail ordered was getting too small and that was the biggest size they had.

And then, it happened. On June 19, 2010, I developed shortness of breath walking a very short distance. I decided I was probably just tired or dehydrated and went home and took a nap. That decision nearly cost me my life.

The next day, on my way to work, the whole house of cards came crashing down. I got out of the car and with each step toward the office door, I began to suffocate. I was breathing in and out as fast as I could, but there was no oxygen to be had. By the time I got near the building, my legs gave out and my skin turned a pale white.

This was the end, I thought. 37 years will be all I get. There in the parking lot, I started to think how disappointing it all was. I was convinced I was dying of a heart attack and wasn't going to live. With the oxygen slowly leaving my body, I decided I had to get help. I fished my phone out of my pocket and somehow called my parents, who had just dropped me off because my car was in the shop.

They came back and got me and took me to the emergency room. While on the way there, barely conscious in the car, my mind started to run wild. Since I knew I was going to die, I started giving my Mom instructions on what to do with my belongings, who to call and how to empty my bank account. Then, I had a thought.

When my parents brought me home from the hospital as a newborn baby, I weighed 6 pounds and 10 ounces. Now they were taking me back to the hospital, 37 years later, and I weighed over 500 pounds. Boy, I really screwed that up. What had I done? I had been given a good life and I wasted it.

We got to the ER and I must have been white as a sheet, or turning blue when I stumbled in. I remember the receptionist saying "Can I help you?" And I remember whispering to her, out of breath "I can't breathe."

I have never seen so many people move so quickly in my life. They had me into a wheelchair, into a room and onto a table in about 30 seconds. I had oxygen, an EKG and an IV started in another 30 seconds.

They continued to run tests. I was in the ER for about 6 hours. A few hours into it, I had to go to the bathroom. So I took off the oxygen mask, went and came back completely out of breath. They checked my blood oxygen level and it had dropped 30 points.

No more going to the bathroom. "You're not going home anytime soon with oxygen levels like that," they told me. Finally, after several hours and more tests the doctor comes in. "We don't think it's your heart, Mr. Ganey. Everything looks good there."

That's a relief. So if not a heart attack, then what? Another doctor will see you soon.

After more time, here comes another doctor, a cardiologist. He ran me through the diagnosis, the tests, explained everything in detail. He was impressive. He said they ruled out the heart and instead suspected blood clots in my lungs.

He didn't have to say any more. I knew what a pulmonary embolism was because I had read about it over the years. The journalist David Bloom died from a pulmonary embolism in 2003 while covering the war in Iraq for NBC. The blood clots develop in your legs and travel to your lungs where they accumulate. If enough of the clots build up, they cut off your oxygen supply and you die instantly.

Except I was lucky. I made it to the hospital on time. I was going to live. I have never felt a greater sense of relief in my life.

But back to the doctor. He told me that what they really needed to do was a CT scan to confirm the blood clots in my lungs, only there was a problem. The machine had a weight limit of 360 pounds and they couldn't do the test. The doctor told me he would admit me and begin treating me for a pulmonary embolism based solely on the best guess he could come up with on what was happening.

Essentially, what he was telling me with the utmost sympathy and sugar coating was this: I was too fat for the machine, so they were doing the best they could. After several hours in the emergency room, I would be admitted.

How long? 2 or 3 days, on the low end. They're going to try to avoid operating. Operating? If the blood clots in my lungs that were suffocating me didn't break up on their own, they would have to cut me open and take them out.

For now, the treatment was blood thinners, or more specifically anti-coagulants. They shot me full of something called Heparin and started a Heparin IV drip, which would last for a week. I must have gone through 20 of those bags. In addition, they started a fairly high dose of Coumadin. This would take a few days to take effect. Coumadin? My grandfather was on that drug for years at the end of his life. I knew it was a powerful drug with awful side effects.

But at least I was going to live.

During my time in the hospital, I met several doctors, 2 nutritionists, specialists...everything. After some more tests, the following became very clear to me:

1.) I came very, very close to dying. I was told 1 in 4 pulmonary embolism victims die within seconds. The first symptom is sudden death. The blood clots form in the legs due to inactivity, travel to the lungs and collect there. This is called Deep Vein Thrombosis (DVT.) The clots clog the main arteries in your lung and cause shortness of breath or worse.

2.) The #1 risk factor for what happened to me was my weight.

3.) I had a choice: lose weight or die. I was told this would keep happening to me. One nurse point blank asked me: "Do you really want to spend the rest of your life in the health care system?"

The week I spent in the hospital was a miserable time. I couldn't do anything without somebody helping me. The low point came when I needed help going to the bathroom. With every limitation, with my increasing lack of mobility, I became more and more enraged at myself.

How did I let it get this bad?

What am I doing?

Is the food really worth it?

Because of the tubes and wires, they wouldn't let me take a shower. That's right, I went one whole week without a shower. As you can imagine, I wanted to kill myself. Also, the nurses would come every few hours to draw blood. Because of my weight, they could never find a vein to draw the blood. I had blood drawn from my hands, my wrist, my fingers...you name it. They couldn't get the IV into my hand and wound up sticking it into my arm, where it became infected.

More limitations. More special treatment. More being told I couldn't do something because of my weight.

And then I snapped. Enough was enough. There would be no more of this.

I drew the line. This is where it would end. I didn't want any more sympathy. There would be no more pity for Bryan Ganey.

I'm only 37, I thought. I've got things to do. There is more to life than eating. I will not go out like this. I will find other things to eat. I will seek out other food, more nutritious food. This all ends now.

And so, I was discharged from the hospital after a week. I weighed 577 pounds. I walked out of that hospital, head held high, absolutely determined not to come back. There would be no more sympathy for Bryan. There would be no more blood clots. There would be no quick fix. All I cared about was getting started.

My message for the medical community was simple: I don't want your pills, I don't want your surgery. All I want is for you to get out of my way.

COMING HOME: NOW WHAT? GETTING STARTED

After being in the hospital for 6 straight days, I had worked myself up to the point that I was determined to do something about my weight problem. I was done. No more. Right before I was released, I got to take my first shower in 6 days. It was heaven. I couldn't really do a very thorough job since there was no detachable shower head (use your imagination,) but it was better than nothing.

I put back on the same clothes I had worn into the emergency room. (A pair of custom-made, size 74 dress slacks and a 7X shirt, both featured in the pictures chapter at the end of this book.) Then I waited for my parents to pick me up.

I thought for several hours about how I could lose weight differently this time. What could I do that would make it last? How do I prevent myself from launching a lifestyle change with great fanfare, only to revert back to the same old behaviors and laziness that got me into trouble in the first place?

But this time will be different. I just almost died.

Then, the first of my own personal "rules" popped into my head:

If it's not forever, it's not worth doing.

In other words, if the change I am making is not one that I am prepared to stick with for the rest of my life, then I am not doing it.

Failure is a great teacher. I had learned in the past that losing a bunch of weight quickly with no plan to keep it off really was worse than not having lost it in the first place. The approach is key.

Think back to the previous times you have lost weight and gained it back. Now accept and realize that every one of those attempts was a failure because it was never going to work in the first place. It wasn't because you were doing it wrong. It wasn't because you didn't stick to it.

It was because the plan was a failure. So with that in mind, I was not going to repeat any of my failures.

Oddly enough, I have said often throughout the last 3 years that a diet is the only consumer product in America where people blame themselves when it doesn't work. We tolerate that from no other manufacturer or service provider.

So now what? How do I focus all of this motivation, drive, desire and fed-upness into a plan of action? I broke it down into a few categories

EATING

I decided from the beginning that I need to eat and I need to eat a lot. I cannot be on an eating plan where I am expected to eat small frozen dinners. I need bulk. I need to feel full. This is where the principle of calorie density comes in handy. What is that?

Essentially, it is the way you evaluate a food. For instance watermelon (as the name implies) is mostly water. It is 9 calories an ounce. The leading brand of nacho cheese tortilla chips is 150 calories per ounce. So, 10 ounces of those chips is 1,500 calories. 10 ounces of the watermelon is 90 calories. Same with green beans. 9 calories an ounce. Bananas are 25 calories an ounce.

In other words, look how much more food you get for calories you are spending. I could go on and on, but I want you to do your own research.

The point is, I need large amounts of food. I need to eat and eat often. So I developed a plan with the assistance of a registered dietitian to do just that.

I decided on 6 meals a day. 3 large, healthy meals and 3 snacks. You may be different, but I am just a big eater and always will be. This has worked for me.

This also meant that I needed to decontaminate my house. When I got home from the hospital, there wasn't any remotely healthy thing to eat in my kitchen. The best I could do for dinner was a plain baked potato, a hamburger patty and some whole kernel corn.

The next day, I threw everything in my kitchen away and went to the store. I bought some things I no longer eat, but I did the best I could. I was (and still am) on a low-fat, low-sodium cardiac diet. It was hard to find foods with any processing that weren't loaded with sodium. Again, I did the best I could.

Remember, there are only 2 things that don't have any calories: water and air. Everything else, measure it and write it down. Even if you overeat…measure it and write it down. Maintain control at all times.

EXERCISE

At 577 pounds, I wasn't exactly going to be out running marathons. In fact, I couldn't do much at all and could barely walk unassisted. I started out pushing the grocery cart around the store, because that gave me something to lean on.

This is where patience comes in. Another of my principles I have lived by the last 3 years has been this:

I don't care how long any of this takes.

Your lifestyle change is so important, it has no end. It doesn't matter how long it takes. You aren't trying to lose a certain amount of weight by a certain time. You are trying to get healthier and live a better life.

So back to the exercise. My lung doctor cleared me for "light walking." Essentially, that meant walking about 3 times a week at about 5 or 10 minutes a day. No problem. I knew that would be the beginning. Over time, I would increase it.

And that is exactly what I did. 5 minutes became 10 minutes became 30 minutes which turned into 3 hours and on and on. I went from pushing a grocery cart around the store to walking to the end of my driveway after a couple months. I eventually progressed to running 5K's and 10K's. But it all began with the walking.

You start where you are because that is the only place you can start.

And finally, another very important thing to think about as you begin your lifestyle change.

I don't care what anyone thinks.

You have got to let go of what other people think. You cannot let it consume you. If you are like I was, I wanted the approval of others. I would obsess about what others thought. This is a guaranteed pathway to lifestyle change failure.

In the end, it is you and only you that can make these changes. You are up against the Great American Way Of Life. There is food everywhere. There are people who will enable you to fail and sabotage any progress you make, 24 hours a day, 7 days a week. You have to watch out for them.

You are changing your lifestyle because you want to live. There is no other reason to be doing it. The road is too long and the work is too hard to do it for any other superficial reason.

Oh, I almost forgot one thing. Unable to cope with the food commercials, I cut my cable and quit watching TV.

This may be unrealistic for you, but it was a necessary step for me. It was just something I had to do.

CHANGING YOUR MINDSET – YOU ARE THE 5%

This is not a diet book. I am not offering you some special plan you can follow to lose 30 pounds in 30 days. I am not going to insult your intelligence by telling you how easy it all is. It isn't. Losing weight is actually quite easy. Keeping it off is the very, very hard part.

You may have heard the statistics, which vary depending on the source. Between 9 and 10 people that lose weight gain it all back. I've read 90%. I've read 95%. It doesn't matter. What really matters is that we have a plan to lose weight that includes another plan to keep it off. If you approach your lifestyle change correctly, you will be the 5% and not the 95%. Say it out loud: I am the 5%.

Early on in this journey, I realized that there was no point to losing weight if I couldn't keep it off. I have been through the depressing emotional trauma of losing a large amount of weight and gaining it all back. It's a terrible feeling. It's also humiliating. There was no way I was going through that again.

Think about that for a minute. That point of view will absolutely change how you approach your lifestyle change. From the outset, think not about losing weight. Think about keeping it off and maintaining a lower weight. If you apply that as a standard, you see why everything and everybody else fails.

Diet food. This is what everybody eats to lose weight and what happens when they stop eating it? They gain all the weight back. Unless you are going to eat boxed dinners you buy off the TV the rest of your life, don't bother.

Pills. At best, diet pills do nothing for you and at worst, they cause very serious health problems. No matter what some doctor on TV says, there is no such thing as a "fat-burning" pill. None of it works, none of it will ever work and your money is going to be wasted. Don't do it.

Low-carb diets. Are you really, honestly going to live on mostly meat the rest of your life? Doubtful, since if you did, you wouldn't live very long. Again, there is no point to attempting any diet plan that you cannot commit to the rest of your life.

So that is the first step. What can you realistically do? Everybody is different. This is where you have to look inside yourself and assess the situation.

Here are a few good first steps to follow.

1.) <u>Get all of your health problems out in the open, on the table.</u>
Men especially, I am talking to you. Pretending you don't have high blood pressure doesn't make it go away. Go to the doctor. Get a full check-up. If you are prescribed medication, take it as directed. If you have problems sleeping, go see a doctor and get a sleep

study done. If you're diagnosed with sleep apnea, follow your doctor's orders and use your CPAP nightly. It will save your life.

2.) <u>Make an appointment with a registered dietitian.</u> Learn about portion control, proper nutrition and eating a balanced diet. Go to the appointment. Take notes and ask lots of questions.

3.) <u>Talk to your doctor about what you're wanting to do.</u> If at any point along the way, any doctor or health professional belittles your desire to better yourself and tells you it can't be done, find another doctor with a better attitude. Yes, 95% may gain all the weight back, but remember...you are the 5%.

4.) <u>Set your expectations correctly.</u> This is going to take years. That's right; I said it. If your goal is to lose 20 pounds by your family reunion, don't buy this book. I don't want your money. There are plenty of other gimmicks and diets on the bookshelf for you to try. My plan is simple: long-term weight loss is not only the goal, it is the only goal. You would be better off losing 50 pounds in the first year and keeping it off than you would be losing 100 pounds the first year and gaining back 200. Studies have shown the longer it takes to lose weight, the more likely the person is to keep that weight off.

5.) <u>Weigh once and then put the scale away.</u> Yes, you need a starting weight. If you're extremely overweight like I was, there may not be a scale that can accurately weigh you. I had to weigh at one point on a truck scale. But I wanted that starting weight. But after you get that beginning weight, put the scale away for 1 month. That's right, I am telling you not to weigh on a scale for a month. When most people begin a diet, they race from one weigh-in to the next, worshiping the scale. They become obsessed with pleasing the scale. It all becomes about moving that number at all costs. No consideration is given to your health, new habits being formed or your lifestyle being permanently changed. That is the diet mindset. The problem is eventually the diet will end, you'll lose interest and be unable to keep up that extreme approach. So don't do it.

Again: weigh once and put the scale away. Your goal here is to improve your health and live a better life, not win a weight loss contest. You will see this repeated over and over in this book, because that is how important I think it is.

6.) <u>The food that you will eat will come from the grocery store.</u> If you haven't been in awhile, you might have to ask somebody where it is. Take a friend, learn how it works. Once you park your car, there will be a grocery cart you can use to collect your items. In some parts of the country, this is called a "buggy" or a "shopping cart" or if you live in the UK, a "trolley." Some of you haven't been to the grocery store since you were 14 years old. You're going to be spending a lot of time there, so familiarize yourself with it. **Warning:** the grocery store can be a dangerous place as well. It is loaded with as much junk food as a fast food restaurant. However, I will teach you to know the difference and only buy the good stuff.

7.) <u>Say goodbye to restaurants, vending machines, drive-thrus, pizza delivery, coffee shops, donuts at the office...all of it.</u> This is the new you. Do whatever you have to do: have a funeral, write a letter to yourself, whatever. But it's over. These are not healthy sources of food for you and won't be in the future.

8.) <u>But wait...no more restaurants...ever?</u> Before I lose you completely, hear me out. A long time ago, perhaps when you were a child, restaurants were considered a treat. Dining out was reserved for special occasions only. Then sometime in the last 20-30 years or so, it became the alternative to cooking at home. Now it has turned into the only way to eat for a lot of people. This is a disaster. You cannot surrender your lifestyle change to a restaurant, whose only goal it is to sell you as much food as possible, as cheaply as possible.

So will you be able to go to a restaurant again someday? Yes, you will. But not for now. More on that later in the book.

9.) <u>Yes, you are going to need to exercise.</u> However, unless you are a qualified personal trainer, all you know about exercise is what you've seen on TV and that is the incorrect way to exercise. Do not be one of these people that joins the gym, goes for 2 weeks straight, works out like a maniac, hurts themselves and then is never seen or heard from again. That is, until you run into them at the buffet. Ever wonder how gyms make their money? The majority of the people who belong simply donate their dues monthly and do not use the facility. Joining a gym is probably not something you will do for awhile.

10.) <u>Prepare to eat and eat all the time.</u> Food is not a reward, food is not a celebration, food is not for pleasure, food is not happiness, food is not comfort. Food is fuel. Nothing more, nothing less. You eat because you have to. And to be healthy, you need to eat healthy food regularly. Whether or not you are hungry has nothing to do with it. You need a lot of food when you wake up in the morning. Then you need more food a few hours later, then lunch, then some more food a few hours after that, then dinner, then an evening snack. You are going to eat 3 meals per day and 3 snacks. Starvation is not an option. You are what you eat. The 95% that gain the weight back ride the roller coaster of frozen diet dinners, meal replacement shakes, protein bars, diet pills and other assorted nonsense. Again, you are the 5%. You are only going to make changes you can live with for the rest of your life.

THE MENTAL BLOCK

For 37 years, I literally spent hours, days, weeks months and years with a mental block about my weight. Anyone who has ever struggled with their weight will be familiar with some of these thoughts, which used to run through my mind constantly:

"I could never do that." This is what I would think when I would see someone who had successfully lost weight or was losing weight. I could never do that. I can't. It's impossible. I just can't. Let's break this statement down a little further.

Whatever "that" is that you've decided you can't do, you're probably right. Most people that lose weight do so through dangerous or unhealthy means. So stop comparing yourself to everybody else. When you lose weight, you're going to go about it the right way. You're going to do it your way, not their way. Everybody is different. What works for one person is not likely to work for another. You want a customized solution to your weight issue. As for what everybody else is thinking or doing: like my mother always used to tell me, YOU worry about YOU. Forget what everybody else is doing.

I'm also reminded of the "I could never do that" syndrome when I am working out at the gym. There is always going to be somebody that is stronger, faster, better when it comes to working out. I had to learn that what anyone else is doing has no bearing on what I am doing. Physical ability is person-specific. I am 40 years old and have bad knees. I just lost nearly 400 pounds. So what if I can't lift as much as the other guy in the gym. Who cares! This is about you, no one else.

"I'll do it next year." A new year. New beginnings, new possibilities. This sets off perhaps the greatest yearly waste of time in our lives: the new year's resolution.

I've done it so many times. Each year, I would pig out for 2 months straight at the holidays, all justifying it with that eye on the artificial January 1 deadline. I actually convinced myself that as soon as the clock struck midnight on New Year's Eve, I would magically start eating right and start going to the gym.

Sure, I would go to the gym....and that gym sure would be full. But by about the 3rd week in January, the gym would be empty and I would be back in the fast-food drive-through. So from my vast experience in failure, I'd like to offer some suggestions to the new year's resolution crowd.

Instead of getting your hopes up that you are going to somehow magically turn your life around based on the calendar, take an honest assessment of your lifestyle. Forget losing a certain amount of weight by a certain time. If you have a lot of weight to lose like I did, the weight isn't the problem. That word "lifestyle" encompasses many things. Our lifestyle is how we live our lives, including:

-How much stress we are under

-The quality of our relationships

-How much sleep we get on a daily basis

-Our overall happiness level with our lives

-The quality and frequency of the meals we eat

-How much physical activity we get on a daily basis

My weight problem was just a symptom of an unhealthy lifestyle. What I ate and how much I ate was just one part of that. I've realized this as I've had a chance to reflect on my life and try to figure out why I overeat, what triggers it, what I can do differently, etc.

So for this year, resolve to look at the big picture. And if you must make a resolution, make an actual resolution that you can follow through on. Something like "I am going to pack my lunch and eat it every day." Or how about "I am going to walk 15 minutes a day, 3 times a week."

If I've learned one thing in all of this, it's that if you cannot do it for the rest of your life, it's not worth doing. Sure, you might be able to work out 10 times a week in the gym and lose 50 pounds in 3 months, but what about the long-term? What about the disappointment that will come when you burn out and can no longer maintain that maniacal level of exercise?

Instead of setting yourself up for that unhappy crash back to reality, take the long view. Don't count on making any changes you cannot maintain for the rest of your life. There is no "next year," there is only right now.

"If I could just _____, then I know I would lose weight." This used to be my specialty and is one of the many gateway statements into the magical kingdom of denial.

First of all, if/then thinking almost never comes true. To illustrate this example, apply it to something else in your daily life. "If my child would stop misbehaving, then I wouldn't be so stressed out." The truth is, the kid is always going to act up and you have to decide (or not decide) whether or not you're going to be stressed out. In other words, you control your reaction.

By saying you have to be able to do something else in order to lose weight, you're employing a delaying tactic. What you're really saying to yourself is "I am not ready to handle this problem right now."

AND THERE IS NOTHING WRONG WITH THAT.

There, I have said it. Your eyes do not deceive you. I actually told you there is nothing wrong with not being ready to lose weight. It took me 37 years to work up to the mindset and achieve the focus and controlled intensity to be able to pull this off. It shouldn't have taken me 37 years to get to this point, nor should it for you. Now I'm not saying it's OK to put off doing something about your health. If you are extremely overweight like I was, your health is threatened every minute of every day. If the house is on fire, you get out. Having a sense of urgency about it is key.

But let's not pretend here. I don't believe people are really ever "fat and happy," but they can be content. Sure, being overweight means you don't fit in the clothes you want to fit in. But you can always buy bigger clothes. Maybe you think being overweight means you aren't as attractive. But you know what? There will always be people who find other overweight people attractive. I had girlfriends when I was well over 500 pounds. So you can become very content. I was miserable, but I was content.

The point is, if you're not ready, you're not ready. Be honest about that. Which leads me to the next great lie we tell ourselves.

"I can't find the motivation to lose weight." After I lost 250 pounds in 1997 and 1998 in 14 months, I spectacularly dove head-first off the wagon and gained all of it back in about 9 months. It was

humiliating and depressing. That failure was so traumatic that it plunged me into a deep, dark depression for the next 12 years.

Only it didn't have to be that way.

I came to realize that my approach and method back then was doomed to failure from the start. But it had a harmful consequence, beyond just me gaining the weight back that one time. I bought into the "lightning bolt" theory of weight loss. I thought that I had lost all that weight before because out of nowhere came a lightning bolt, a shock to the system, an epiphany, a realization, a magical force that would motivate me to lose weight.

Sorry, the truth is it doesn't work that way in the real world. And you don't want it to work that way.

Inspiration and motivation can come from somewhere else, it can get you started. Like in my case. I almost died from a pulmonary embolism. I spent a miserable week in the hospital, ready to kill myself over my circumstance. But that experience helped me to get started. What keeps me going is a much deeper desire to have a better life.

Real motivation to lose weight comes from deep down inside of us. You want to live longer. You want to be healthier. You're tired of dreading going to the doctor. You're tired (like I was) of all the pills. You don't want any more sympathy. You want to live to see your kids graduate high school. You want to live to see your grandchildren grow up. One of my favorite things to do is make lists. Go ahead and try it. Get a legal pad and a pen and write "reasons to lose weight" at the top of it. Write out the reasons by your own hand. No smartphone apps, no tablets, no computers. Just you writing. Look at what you've written. Think about it. Stare at the page. Spend time in a quiet place with your list with just you and no other distractions. THAT is the motivation to lose weight, my friend.

If you have a mental block about your weight loss like I did, you have to overcome it. But how you overcome it is very important. You don't want to waste valuable energy and motivation on stupid diets or methods. For this to last, you have to do it right. Let's break it down a little further.

Stop trying to lose weight. No, your eyes do not deceive you. I just told you to stop trying to lose weight. Stop thinking in terms of your weight as being the sole, chief motivator in all of this. The goal should be instead to pursue a healthier lifestyle, one of the many benefits of which is a lower body weight. "Losing weight" is a short-term goal that will not last by itself.

Think in terms of years, not days, weeks or months. When I was trying to overcome my mental block, it helped me to think of what I was doing in a much longer-term. The result was I was able to break the boom and bust diet cycle and adopt habits and behaviors that will lead to a more permanent lifestyle change. Remember: if you are not going to do it forever, there is no point to doing it.

And now a final point about the mental block. The only way to overcome the mental block is to just start. The way to start your lifestyle change is the familiar marketing slogan from a famous shoe company: just do it.

There is no dramatic start. There is no fanfare. Just eat a healthy breakfast and go for a walk.

BREAKING ALL THE RULES: WEIGHT LOSS MYTHS

Myth: "I don't eat that much."

This used to be one of my favorites. Truth is, you may not eat a large quantity of food, but if what you're eating is very high in calories, you will be overweight. We are what we eat. I used to regularly eat 10,000 calories a day. It's no wonder I weighed 577 pounds. Denial is a powerful force that will only hold you back.

The bottom line: if you are overweight, you really are eating that much.

Myth: Eating in the car, eating in front of the television, or eating in front of the computer is wrong and you're a bad person for doing it.

I always enjoy reading this one. I am pleased to report it is complete nonsense. In the last 3 years, I have lost nearly 400 pounds committing the following sins, according to the "experts:" I eat breakfast every day in front of the computer. I snack all day at work in front of a computer. I eat dinner and watch TV at the same time. Sometimes I eat dinner, watch TV and surf the Internet, all at the same time. That's talent, right?

I eat in the car. I eat and drive at the same time. Sometimes I eat in the grocery store parking lot, right from the food package. This whole idea that we should only eat at the dining room table is a complete fantasy in this day and age. I don't even have a dining room table (that I know of.)

It's not where you're eating your food, it's what you're eating and how many calories you're consuming. Trying to follow unrealistic rules about where you should eat takes your eye off the ball. It's a popular rule, however, because humans are addicted to making things more complicated than they need to be.

The bottom line: Mindless eating can occur anywhere. As long as you know how much you're eating and you keep track of it, you can eat anywhere.

Myth: Eating at night is bad and will make you fat.

If eating at night made you fat, I would still weigh 577 pounds. The truth is, I eat around the clock. As long as the total amount I am consuming is right for me, it doesn't matter when I eat it.

Sometimes I eat dinner at 5pm. Sometimes I eat it at 9pm. I've had dinner at 11pm.

I once woke up at 2 in the morning so ravenously hungry, I could've eaten the wallpaper off the walls. I made myself a bowl of oatmeal with a piece of fruit and ate it. And you know what? I still lost weight that week. I just added it to my food diary for that day, ate the food and went back to bed. And lived to tell about it. Imagine that!

But...doesn't everything you eat turn to fat if you go right to bed after you eat it? No, it doesn't. Think about the nonsense of this oft-repeated statement. If I eat an apple, which has practically zero fat, how is that going to turn to fat in my stomach just because I am asleep? Please.

The bottom line: As long as the total calories of what you're eating doesn't exceed your requirements for that day, eating at night will not make you fat.

Myth: To lose weight, I have to starve myself. I can eat no more than 1,500 calories.

I don't know about you, but I could never get by on 1,500 calories a day. The truth is, everybody's calorie requirements are different. It all depends on how much physical activity you engage in during the day. Somebody that sits at a desk all day won't be able to eat as much as say, a delivery driver who runs up and down stairs all day.

Starvation is one of the biggest reasons I believe people fail at weight loss. They completely overdo it trying to pursue a quick fix, get discouraged and quit. This is very sad. Only eating 1,500 calories a day is as extreme as trying to work out in the gym 20 times a week is. It's not sustainable.

There are different calorie calculators available online and there are differing methods for determining the appropriate number of calories you should consume. Factors such as your desired goal weight, age, height, activity level, etc. all play a part.

For myself, in the beginning, I was eating 1,500-1,600 calories a day. When I boosted that to 2,400 calories, I started losing weight faster. I believe it was because my body was in starvation mode, conserving resources instead of using them. It worked for me. Everybody is different.

The bottom line: you need food to live. You can starve yourself or stop eating to lose weight temporarily, but only for so long.

Myth: If I work out twice a day, 14 times a week, I can eat whatever I want.

Exercise is very important and is absolutely essential to your lifestyle change. However, exercise has a very lousy return when it comes to weight loss. For example, for every 100 calories burned, you have to run a mile. One bad trip through the drive-thru is 1,000 calories.

The bottom line: you cannot out-exercise your stupidity. Exercise is central to a healthy body and a healthy mindset. But unless you're Michael Phelps, weight is lost at mealtime, not in the gym.

Myth: I know someone who eats like a horse and magically still stays skinny.

Sorry, no you don't. And here's why. Yes, you may see this mythical thin person eat a large amount of food. But do you really know how much they eat all day? Are you tracking their calories and their exercise? What do they do for a living? Perhaps they just eat one large meal per day and that is what you witnessed.

The bottom line: the math is the math. No one escapes it. There is no magical, mythical skinny person that defies the laws of nature. They don't exist. This is what we tell ourselves to make ourselves feel like victims and feel better about overeating.

Myth: Everything In Moderation

It has been said that you can eat anything you want as long as you just eat it in moderation. There are a few problems with this. If you are significantly overweight, it is safe to say that you cannot do anything in moderation and this strategy has failed you. A famous commercial for a famous snack food product says you can't eat just one. There is a reason for this. The "food" is engineered to make you want it. As a food addict, I can tell you that for many things, 1 is too many and 100 is never enough.

The bottom line: "everything in moderation" doesn't work because "everything" is not moderation.

Myth: There Are No Bad Foods

You can have anything you want, right? I will answer that question with a question: how has that strategy worked out for you so far? Consider this: a banana is approximately 25 calories per ounce. A popular candy bar that claims to cure hunger is 135 calories per ounce. What is going to fill you up more? A half a candy bar or a large banana?

The bottom line: some foods simply offer no nutritional value and should be avoided. You cannot reprogram your taste buds to like healthy food by continuing to have "just a little" of the processed garbage that made you overweight in the first place.

Myth: I know what works, I'll just do it again.

The definition of insanity is doing the same thing over and over again and expecting a different result. If you have lost weight before and not kept it off, that approach was a failure. It should not be repeated because the failure will be repeated. Unlike the stock market, past performance is indeed an indicator of future results. You must study your failures and not repeat them.

The bottom line: the goal is not to lose weight. The goal is to keep it off. There is a difference and we will talk more about that later.

Myth: Eating Healthy Is Expensive. You need to eat special foods to lose weight.

This myth got started by people buying diet foods at the grocery store. The "light" and "fat-free" versions of processed foods do indeed cost more than the full fat versions. But that garbage isn't going to be what you're eating.

In addition, people who eat in restaurants 5 and 10 times a week will get on a health kick, go to the grocery store, spend $200 and then proclaim "eating healthy is expensive!" I know this is true because I have seen me do it.

If you stop eating at restaurants, stop buying mostly processed food and instead buy fruits, vegetables, whole grains, lean meats and low-fat dairy, you will discover eating healthy is quite inexpensive.

I came across a news story that talks about how eating healthy costs more and since the economy is so bad, darn it, some people just won't be able to afford the extra cost. So I guess I should just give up, crawl back into my cave and go back to eating cheeseburgers, snack cakes and ramen noodles every 5 minutes.

Are you kidding me? Really? What nonsense. The reason this is a complete lie is because the article does not address the #1 cause of unhealthy eating:

Eating out all the time.

Even if you accept the premise that healthy grocery shopping costs more than unhealthy grocery shopping (which I don't, by the way) it's still cheaper to eat healthy than not if you stay out of the restaurants. Let's look at the math:

According to an article on the Internet, the average American spends $2,736 a year in restaurants and bars. That's an average of about $50 a week. For most people I know, it's more. But whatever.

The article says eating healthy costs an extra $7.28 a week. I think if you quit eating out, you can afford the $7.28.

And what about other sources of unhealthy eating? How about the vending machines? Your daily drive-thru latte purchase? It all adds up.

Say nothing of the impact on your health. What about the financial consequences of an unhealthy diet, such as more doctor visits and more medications? How much does that cost?

The bottom line: eating healthy does NOT cost more. Unhealthy eating does.

Myth: Don't eat too many carbohydrates.

Nonsense. It's all about the calories, not the carbs. I eat bread, oatmeal, rice, potatoes, spaghetti and other assorted carbs in large quantities. According to the logic of the anti-carb crowd, I should weigh 1,000 pounds.

The bottom line: If you have a medical condition that requires you to limit and track your carbohydrate intake, like being diabetic, then you absolutely have to count your carbs. Otherwise, just another myth.

Myth: You need special pills or a patch to lose weight.

I have lost nearly 400 pounds in 3 years and have never once taken a diet pill. I have come to realize they are a complete waste of money. But they are popular because people want the quick fix. They want something else to do the work for them. Sorry, it's never going to happen.

The bottom line: unless prescribed by a doctor, diet pills are a waste of money and can be dangerous. Oh, and the only way the weight loss patch works is if you put it over your mouth.

So there you have it. This has been an overview of several popular weight loss myths. Hopefully you can begin to see that there really is no quick fix and losing weight takes hard work.

Are you ready to change your life? If so, keep reading.

TIME TO CHANGE YOUR LIFESTYLE

What exactly is a "lifestyle change?"

You've probably heard the following saying many times in your life: "It's not a diet, it's a lifestyle change."

What comes to mind is the idea that not only are you changing what you eat and how much, but you're also exercising.

But as I've discovered over the last 3 years, it's much, much more than that. You don't get to be 577 pounds without having several serious problems going on around you. But when it comes to changing that lifestyle, here are just a few things I changed that aren't necessarily just diet and exercise.

1.) Your friends. That's right, your friends. In much the same way that a recovering alcoholic gets rid of their drinking buddies, a food addict has to ditch their "eating buddies." If all you do with somebody is go out to eat, then that relationship is destructive. If the people you hang out with have become a bad influence, time for them to go.

2.) Grocery Shopping. If the junk food isn't in your house, you can't eat it. If you swing open your refrigerator and look inside it, what is available? Is it full of crap? If it is, time to throw it all away and fill it with healthy food. Or the absolute worst, is there nothing in it at all? Time to start grocery shopping...stat. As far as eating out in restaurants goes, this is out of control. It used to be dining out was reserved for special occasions. Now it's turned into 3 and 5 times a week. I believe in order to change your lifestyle, a large percentage of your food has to come from the grocery store.

3.) Your schedule.

Early to bed, early to rise, makes a man healthy, wealthy and wise."
-Benjamin Franklin

I've heard this said all my life, but in the last 3 years, I have realized that it is 100% true. I simply could not have lost nearly 400 pounds on my own without converting to a daytime schedule. And I will never work any other schedule, ever again.

There is something about going to bed early that instills discipline. Getting up early is refreshing, energizing and puts me in a completely different frame of mind than sleeping until noon does.

In addition, night time promotes all of the demons. Darkness. Being alone. Brightly lit fast food restaurant signs. Late night pizza delivery. Endless TV watching.

To anyone considering a lifestyle change, I would absolutely say switching to a day shift as soon as humanly possible is a total must. This may just be unique to me, but I'll include it anyway. Part of my cycle of self-destruction included working a night schedule. I would get off work, then stay up all night watching TV and binging on junk food. By the time I fell asleep at 4 or 5 in the morning, I was stuffed with thousands of calories. For me, it took switching to an early morning shift to help jump-start my healthy lifestyle change. It turns out it is true what Benjamin Franklin said. Except for the wealthy part, all of that has come true for me. (And some may argue the wise part.)

4.) Television. I almost never watch TV anymore. In fact, I've thought of giving it away. What's on TV, anyway? Non-stop food commercials. I used to watch the food shows all the time. But I have discovered that I can't anymore. Everything they show is one gigantic eating trigger. I used to think I had to watch certain TV shows...that there is no way I could live without the TV. Turns out I don't need it at all.

Your lifestyle is your life. If you want to change your lifestyle, you're going to have to change your life. After 3 years of doing this, I can tell you this: it is very hard. But as the saying goes, it is difficult, but not impossible.

Think of it this way: if you want to lose weight, all of your habits, behaviors, food that you eat, body movements, all of it contribute to your current state of health.

To make that change, to improve your health, requires the modification of habits, behaviors, food that you eat and body movements.

What makes this a very tall order is none of it will last unless you do it forever. The problem with all of that is that for many of us (myself included, before June 20, 2010) food has become a reward. Food has become entertainment. Food has become happiness.

That all has to go out the window. Food is fuel. Nothing more. The thin person does not have a problem with this. They are perfectly capable of (for now) celebrating with food, eating foods high in sugar, fat, salt and calories in small portions and getting by.

But not us. Not me. Not other heavy people. We've gone too far. We can't do it. We can't stop.

Which is why we can never start.

Back to changing the lifestyle. There are so many traditions and things that we do where unhealthy food is ingrained into our routines. To be successful, long-term, I believe it all has to go.

Used to eating concession food at the movies? Bring your own healthy alternatives.

Used to eating hotdogs and nachos at the baseball game? Bring your own better food.

Eat out of the vending machines at work? Don't. Pack your own lunch and snacks.

That's what has to happen. Those key behaviors have to be changed. And that's why it's hard.

But you can do it! If I can, anyone can. And that's the truth.

I get asked all the time: "How can I lose weight like you did? How do I find the motivation to lose X number of pounds? Will you tell me what to eat?"

As well-intentioned as those questions are, they all miss the point completely. Simply losing weight should never be the focus. As a matter of fact, it's a counterproductive way to think. Being overweight is a symptom of an unhealthy lifestyle, it is not the cause of it.

Before you start thinking about losing weight and trying to add years to your life and life to your years, you have to be in the proper frame of mind. You need to think about how you can make your lifestyle change permanent. If all you're going to do is temporarily change what you do in order to lose 50 pounds for a wedding and then put it all back on, you may as well not bother.

No, dear reader, what you want is a total lifestyle change. Nothing less will do. That is the best chance you have at getting healthier, losing weight and keeping it off and staying out of the doctor's office. So what are the steps that go into this? First, you have to analyze your own behavior. You know yourself better than anyone else, right?

Identify what your demons are and stay away from them....forever. For me, one of my biggest demons is restaurants. When I am being served food in a restaurant, I cannot control myself. It is very much like an alcoholic in a bar. So I stay far, far away. For you, it might be something simple like mindless eating. Whatever it is, identify it and don't do it!

You can do it. You know you can and so do I. Take your life back. Take it back starting right now.

When it comes to a lifestyle change, how you approach it, the expectations you set are almost more important than the journey itself. I'll give you some examples.

"I need to lose weight" needs to become "I need to adopt a healthy lifestyle, one of the benefits of which is having a lower body weight." See how that works?

"I need to lose 20 pounds by July" needs to become "I'd like to be in shape in time for July. By adopting a healthy lifestyle, that will help me."

Again, if just losing weight is the focus, then give up now. The failure rate on weight loss-based dieting is about 95%. That's 190 out of 200 people gaining it all back.

Don't put yourself through that.

Instead, try this. Don't put a time limit on your lifestyle change.

Don't weigh yourself all the time. Stop wanting it all now, now, now.

When I started my journey, I had a doctor tell me it would take 3 years to lose all this weight. And he might be right. He then suggested weight loss surgery. But I knew, for me, that weight loss surgery wasn't going to fix my problem.

It wasn't going to fix my food addiction problem, only I could do that.

It wasn't going to teach me how to eat right, only I could do that.

It wasn't going to teach me to exercise, only I could do that.

Instead of "I need to lose weight," focus on "I need to maintain a healthier weight."

Because I can tell you from experience, there is *zero* point in losing a bunch of weight if you can't keep it off. Absolutely a waste of time.

How to Handle Negativity

There are going to be people that are not going to want you to change your life. Negativity is everywhere.

We're all guilty of it. You've heard the phrase "misery loves company?" It's very true.

But when it comes to saving your own life and changing your lifestyle, negativity has no place. It must be banished forever and not be tolerated in any way, shape or form. Your mindset on a daily basis is critical to your success.

So what kind of negativity am I talking about?

Sabotage. Face it, some people like us the way we are. People don't like change. Perhaps your partner thinks you'll leave them if you lose weight. Maybe somebody close to you enjoys putting you down because they can't do it themselves. Either way, watch out for sabotage. People always offering you food, for instance, trying to tempt you and enable you into failure. I've run into it before and I simply confront it head-on: "I appreciate the offer, but I am never eating that. Thank you though."

Put-downs. Don't stand for it. This takes many forms, but the basic thrust is the person putting you down doesn't think you can do what you're doing. Or perhaps they can't do it themselves, so they put you down to make themselves feel better. The code words and phrases for the putter-downer are things like "you need to be realistic" and "you can't do this on your own." Again, just like with the sabotage, shut them down: "I am changing my life and I would appreciate you being more supportive."

Fatism. It is an absolute irrefutable fact that the last acceptable form of discrimination in our society is the mistreatment of the overweight. I will debate this issue with anyone who cares to try. It isn't right, but a large portion of society sees big people as less than a human being, if they see them at all. I've experienced this first hand. When I weighed 577 pounds, many people wouldn't even say hello to me. Now they're my best friend. But what they don't realize is I have a mental list and they're on it. So don't tolerate it from your friends and family. You are due the same respect any other person is and don't tolerate the jokes, the put-downs or the comments. You are on a mission to change your life and you will leave the doubters behind.

And one more note about people. Early on, I realized that just like an alcoholic has to ditch their drinking buddies to get clean, I had to do the same thing with my eating buddies. I don't mean to sound drastic, but it had to be done.

When you change your lifestyle, you are changing your life. You are becoming a different, healthier person. That goes for the mind and the body. Your transformation will be the result of your own positive energy and anyone that is not on board with that 100% has to go.

THE 4 STEPS TO SUCCESSFUL, LONG-TERM WEIGHT MANAGEMENT

Step 1: Get Professional Help

Before you begin any lifestyle change, the first thing you must do is talk to your doctor. I used to avoid going to the doctor and it almost cost me my life. You must make an appointment with your doctor and get all of your health problems on the table and address them. I had high blood pressure and wasn't always taking my medication. I had undiagnosed sleep apnea. I was pre-diabetic. My health was a disaster. But I needed to go to the doctor and have all of those conditions properly treated before I could take a single first step. You must go to the doctor. Have a full physical done and see where you stand. Get all the cards on the table, face-up. No more lying to yourself.

Talk to your doctor about what you're wanting to do. Show him or her this book. Explain you want to begin eating 3 well-balanced meals a day and 3 snacks. Ask what exercise you can be cleared for. If you're as large as I was, exercise was very limited to just light walking and sitting and standing. Anything more and I would've injured myself. You have got to be careful. DO NOT start any lifestyle change without consulting your doctor first and getting their approval.

Next, see a registered dietitian. Visit the Academy of Nutrition and Dietetics online (formerly the American Dietetic Association) at EatRight.org. Find a registered dietitian and go see them. It is very important to let go of the lies about diets and quick fixes and embrace the truth: only common sense will set you free. There are many ways to lose weight, but only one way to keep it off: common sense. A good registered dietitian will teach you about portion control and making better choices. I met with a registered dietitian before I got started and it really helped me. Find one and go. Show them this book. Explain what you are trying to do.

Lastly, seek out a qualified personal trainer. Most people "go to the gym" and work out like a maniac for a few weeks, then either injure themselves or burn themselves out. Then they never come back. I see it every year at my gym. Come the first of the year, the gym is jam-packed with everyone making their New Year's resolutions to get healthy. Then after a few weeks, fewer people. By March 1, it's a ghost town. Don't allow this to be you. Remember, if you learn nothing at all from everything I have written, YOU MUST MAKE IT LAST. There is no other way.

The first thing I learned about exercising is that "no pain, no gain" is incorrect. If exercise is causing you pain, you should stop. The point of exercise is to exert yourself just a little bit more than the time before. If you are almost 600 pounds like I was, this means just walking will create exertion. You start where you are. Another thing I learned is that you need days off from working out. More is not always better. I go to the gym 3 times a week, with a day off in between. No more. My body needs time to recover and heal from the workout the time before. I also only work out about an hour each time. Having a personal training program is absolutely worth every penny. Even if you can only consult a trainer every few weeks, you need somebody to help you manage your workout regime.

Step 2: Be Honest With Yourself

Before you get started on your lifestyle change (delete the word "diet" from your vocabulary,) you need to take a personal inventory of your situation. This involves doing something most of us don't do very often, which is being honest with ourselves.

When I was in the hospital at almost 600 pounds, I had a lot of time to think. This period of self-reflection was very important to my success. Ask yourself questions like:

Why do I overeat? Has it always been this way? Was there something specific that took place in my life around the same time I began to get heavy? Look at old pictures of yourself and investigate the time line to get more information about yourself.

How do I eat now? What is the cycle? Analyze the habits and behaviors you are engaging in that are causing you to be at the weight you're at. In my case, 2 of the key habits I had were staying up all night and eating fast food 2 and 3 times a day. When we're honest with ourselves and write it all down and make a list, the denial will start to fade away.

Denial is a powerful force. I used to say and I hear others in a similar situation say that they "don't eat that much." Yes, we really do eat that much. People are too heavy because they eat too much of the wrong things and move their bodies too little. That is an absolute, indisputable, true and pure fact.

The next step in being honest with yourself is to forget about all of the diet failure in your past. I cannot tell you how many people I know that recycle diet failure because "it worked before." Unless you have kept the weight off, THE DIET HAS NOT WORKED. It has BEEN A FAILURE and will continue to be a failure, so STOP

DOING IT. Any fool can lose weight, keeping it off is why you bought this book in the first place. There is absolutely no point in losing weight if you can't keep it off. None. You are better off not having lost a single ounce than you are losing a bunch of weight and rapidly gaining it all back (and more.)

Step 3: Detox

When I think about the difference between how I eat today and how I ate before I went to the hospital several years ago, it is quite a change.

But it has taken a long time to get here.

I think it's rare that anyone could just flip the switch overnight, walking away from a diet of highly processed sugar, salt and fat and into a more healthy one. Your entire palate, all your life, has gotten very used to intense flavors. Your taste buds are expecting that salt, sugar or fat rush with every bite.

If food can be an addiction, and I believe it can be, with myself as an addict...then there has to be a way to go from terrible to healthy. So, like an addict trying to stop abusing a drug, it's time to go through detox. How do you do it? Very carefully.

This is the part where wanting all of the success right now has to fall by the wayside. Remember: you're in this for the rest of your life. You want long-term results, not a quick fix that is going to last a few months.

Forget about losing weight. Time to start re-programming your body to live on and want healthy food. Time to start the detox.

At this stage of the game, the foods that you eat are probably not going to be what you eventually wind up eating. What you drink will not be what you wind up drinking. But you are trying to come down off a very bad trip. Think of this as nutritional methadone.

Also forget about how much you're eating. Again, the focus is on creating new behavior patterns that will last. You may even overeat at this point. It doesn't matter. It's all about being satisfied with the good stuff.

Drinking Water
Somehow, some way, you have to start drinking water. In the beginning, I mixed all my water with sugar-free drink mixes. Also, you can buy fruit-flavored waters. If you must, switch to caffeine-free, sugar-free colas. Whatever it takes to get you from drinking soda all the time to drinking water all the time, you need to get there.

Eating Often
If you eat anything like I used to, it could be a cycle of starving and bingeing. That is, you don't eat breakfast then you wait all the way until you are ravenously hungry, then overeat. This is a big problem. You have got to space out your meals and your eating. What worked for me is eating roughly 6 times a day, about 2 hours between meals: Breakfast, Mid-Morning Snack, Lunch, Mid-Afternoon Snack, Dinner, Evening Snack. That's it. 3 Meals and 3 Snacks. Every day, day in and day out.

Eat In Bulk
The problem with processed foods high in fat, sugar and salt is they are not very filling. You wind up taking in a large number of calories and don't feel full. The goal now is to fill yourself up on food that will make you feel very full, but not have anywhere near the calories of the garbage. This means foods high in fiber, such as oatmeal, high-fiber wheat bread, fruits, vegetables, whole wheat pasta, etc. need to be worked into your diet as much as possible.

Substitutions
One of the big substitutions I made was non-fat yogurt and frozen fruit taking the place of ice cream. I can eat frozen fruit until I am ready to burst, and yet it's only a few hundred calories. I eat Egg

Beaters instead of eggs. Make your own pizzas. Your own healthy burgers. Find creative ways to make better versions of what you used to eat.

And one last thing. Detoxing from an unhealthy lifestyle is going to have its own side effects. You are bound to be cranky, aggravated, mad at the world and very, very unhappy. This is normal. I went through junk food and caffeine withdrawal in the hospital for a week and it was pure misery.

It could take you a couple weeks to detox, maybe even a month. But it's worth it. You just can't give up.

Step Four: Write It Down

Sometimes people will e-mail me or come up to me in person and tell me they're "only" eating 1,200 calories or some ridiculously small amount and they're not losing weight.

Unless the person telling me this weighs 100 pounds and is 4 feet tall, there is only one explanation for their predicament:

They're lying.

I know, I know. They might be lying without knowing their lying. So we'll just say they're lying to themselves, which is the worst sort of lie. Here's the problem with somebody who tells you they're eating 1,200 to 1,500 calories a day and not losing any weight. It's mathematically impossible.

Here is the truth behind the lie. To be a successful calorie counter, you need two things that the liar almost never does:

You must write down everything you eat. Everything that goes into your mouth goes on that paper and is totaled at the end of the day.

You must weigh or measure your portions and count the servings. There can be no exception to this. Because without knowing how many calories you're eating, you have no idea what to write down. Sorry, "about" doesn't cut it.

The liar also tends to conveniently "forget" free food at work, trips to the vending machine, their morning coffee drive-thru run (which can be hundreds of calories, depending) or food served to them by someone else. If somebody else makes the food, how do you know what's in it?

So I tell people to write it down. And then they bring me their food journal. People are ridiculous when it comes to food journaling at first, because they want to lose 100 pounds overnight. So you get something that looks like this:

Breakfast - A cup of coffee and a piece of toast - 100 calories

Snack - 1 Breath Mint, 10 calories

Lunch - A protein Bar, 300 calories

Snack 2 - Plain air-popped popcorn, 100 calories

Dinner - 1 frozen diet dinner, 300 calories

Snack 3 - 1 Cheese stick and a glass of water, 90 calories

Total - 900 calories, and I'm not losing any weight

Now, I will use my powers of perception and ability to read between the lines and tell you what's really going on. Let's examine what this person's food journal probably really should look like:

Breakfast - A cup of coffee and a piece of toast - 100 calories

Peppermint-flavored iced coffee with whipped cream from the coffee drive-thru - 530 calories

Lunch - A protein Bar, 300 calories

Random trip to the vending machine, One 20-ounce bottle of soda 290 calories

Lunch 2 - Free pizza at work because of some contest or performance goal being reached, 800 calories. Remember, if the food is free, it doesn't have any calories, right?

Snack 2 - Plain air-popped popcorn, 100 calories

Random trip to the vending machine, One 20-ounce bottle of soda, 290 calories, plus a candy bar, "because I've been good today," 280 calories

Dinner - 1 frozen diet dinner, 300 calories, 1 garden salad topped with full-fat dressing – 300 calories

More Dinner - Left over pizza brought home "because they were going to throw it away" 800 calories

Snack 3 - 1 cheese stick and a glass of water, 90 calories

Actual total: 4,180 calories, and THAT is why you're not losing any weight

So you can see why it is EXTREMELY important to write down EVERYTHING you put in your mouth during the day. Stop lying to yourself and start writing it down!

By the way, both of these eating plans are equally garbage. It is just as bad, if not worse, to eat too little than it is to not eat enough. Look at these two lists. Where are the fruits? The vegetables? The lean meats? The whole grains? The lowfat dairy? The water?

Eat right. Measure. Write it down. Tell the truth to yourself. And you will lose weight. I promise!

THE DISAPPOINTMENT MACHINE

When I first started my journey 3 years ago, I knew from experience not to get addicted to the high that the scale provides when you're first losing weight. You start to have so much success so quickly, you think that's always going to be there.

So I knew that how much I lost or how quickly I lost it wasn't really important. But, I wanted to be able to chart my progress reasonably.

So I weighed once a month.

I know what you're thinking: "Once a month? Are you insane?" Hear me out.

There are simply too many variations in body weight to weigh every day. Or every week. I think once a month is perfect. Here's why: when the weight loss starts to slow down, or isn't as much as it was last time, you will get disappointed, be discouraged and give up. Not gaining any weight from one time to the next is a roaring success, but you will convince yourself that it is failure. And that is a tragedy.

And so here is what I found myself doing the other times I would lose weight: when it wasn't as much as I thought it should be, I would begin to analyze. And over-analyze. And analyze again. I would literally analyze why I didn't lose a half a pound in 3 days to the point that I worked myself up in such a depression I got discouraged. So I was explaining this to my trainer at the gym and he had a perfect description for this line of thinking: "paralysis by analysis."

I would analyze the scale and worship that number to the point that I would be paralyzed into inaction.

So if you're considering a lifestyle change, use the scale carefully. My advice: weigh once when you get started, then once a month after that. Weigh on your own terms, with your own scale, always at the same time of the day, in the same place, under the same circumstances.

The scale can be a tool that leads you to great success and it can also be a weapon that sends you down the slippery slope to failure. In almost every diet I have ever heard about, it goes something like this: you do whatever you do to lose weight, then weigh in.

Most programs have you weigh in once a week. Or some, for maximum idiocy, have you weigh daily. The focus becomes what the scale says. The goal becomes weight loss and nothing else. And that, my friends, is the road to nowhere.

Thee who worships the scale is destined to drown in disappointment. If your goal in becoming healthier is just to lose weight, save yourself the pain and aggravation and just give up now.

Yes, you have to weigh once in awhile to know where you stand.

But getting caught up in the thrill of quick weight loss means you will become intoxicated with the euphoria of constant success. To say you are setting yourself up for failure would be like saying the Titanic had a moisture problem.

So go easy on yourself. It's OK to throw yourself into your lifestyle change and create dramatic results. But don't be addicted to it. Because one day, that weight loss will stall.

Remember, it's about the rest of your life. Not the next weigh-in on some stupid scale. I just know what it's like to gain weight back you have worked so hard to lose and realize you have to take a long-term view. It's not about next week, or next month or even next year. It's about adding 5, 10, 20 or even 30 years onto your life. Living to see your kids grow up. Regaining your mobility or not living with the cloud of diabetes and heart disease hanging over you.

Never forget that the lifestyle change you create for yourself is more important than any single weigh-in. You are becoming someone else, someone healthier and leaving behind the bad habits and disease of the past.

I have seen people successfully lose a lot of weight, be healthier than ever, be on top of the world…until they step on the scale. The almighty scale tells them they haven't lost any more or have gained back a pound or two and suddenly their world comes crashing down.

Think about that. They went from being happier than ever, satisfied and excited about their success one minute to being depressed and wanting to give up the next. Why? All because they stepped on the scale. Don't do it.

I weigh once a month. I have figured out that this completely disarms the "quick fix" mentality. It makes you think long-term. You are no longer rewarded with the instant gratification of a quick win.

You are taught patience. With my method, the scale returns to its rightful place as a tool in your lifestyle change toolbox, not the reason for it.

Still not convinced? Think about how people do it now. They start their diet by weighing on the scale. They weigh every day. But that's also a mistake. Do you realize how much weight can fluctuate? Over the course of one day, your weight can fluctuate by 10 pounds or more. I easily drink a gallon of water a day. That gallon of water weighs a little more than 8 pounds. What if my body decides to retain it? Hello 8-pound gain. What if your "processing schedule" gets backed up? The scale can go up several pounds that way too.

Success on the scale is also a problem too. It becomes addictive. Let's say you weigh once a week, as many "experts" recommend. So there you are, naked on Monday morning standing on your scale. You can hardly believe your eyes! You lost 5 pounds! YES!!! WAY TO GO!!! AWESOME.

So, exactly one week later, you're back on the scale. You "gain" 2 pounds back. Oops. Now what do you do? Call the therapist! Call off work! This is a disaster! Not really. Here's what happens. Most likely, the 5 pound "loss" wasn't really a loss at all. You were probably somewhat dehydrated. Your body weight has "bounced back" a little bit to what it actually is. In other words, you are doing fine, but the weight loss gods are giving you the finger.

Accept the truth: human body weight fluctuates. It can go up or down several pounds over the course of a day, a week or a couple of weeks.

Once a month works because it teaches you discipline. It forces you to think long-term, not short-term. And it has another benefit: you usually lose weight.

I am begging you, pleading with you....when you begin your lifestyle change, weigh once, write down the number and put the scale away. If you can't resist the urge to weigh, then give the scale to a friend or relative to keep at their house. Only ask for it back once a month. I had such a problem with it in the beginning I had to only weigh at the doctor's office. I couldn't control the constant, destructive urge to "see where I was."

Get rid of the scale. The scale is not your friend. It is an enemy you are forced to visit once a month.

JUST SAY NO TO THE FORCE FEEDERS

One of the things I've had to realize as I learned to manage my food addiction is that some people will not take no for an answer.

Well-meaning, good-intentioned, good-hearted people who think they're being nice and doing you a favor when the reality is, they're doing the opposite. Of course, they don't realize this and couldn't be expected to know this.

You know what I'm talking about. The person who wants to buy you lunch to "celebrate" some one thing or another. The person dropping off candy in your office.

If there is one thing I wish I could shout from the mountaintops to the entire world, it would be this: never offer food to a food addict. And if you do, when they say "no thanks," walk away.

If somebody were a recovering alcoholic, you wouldn't try and convince them to have "just one" beer or try a healthy version of alcohol. Or try and convince them that one visit to the bar won't kill them.

I make it from one day to the next by carefully planning out and bringing with me what I am going to eat. It's what I have to do to get by. It's one of the only reasons for my success thus far and the only way it will continue. I need that control to get by.

So about 80% of the people who offer me food take no offense and simply move on when I say "no thanks." Thank you, 80%. I love you.

Then there's the 10% that says "are you sure?" This 10% is semi-persistent, but gives up after the second "no thanks."

And then there are the people I call the "force feeders." The final 10%. The force feeders will stop at nothing to get you to eat the food they want to make/buy/bring for you.

Declining doesn't get me anywhere with these people. They never give up. In the end, my answer remains the same, but somebody's feelings are always going to get hurt.

So why am I so inflexible? Because it works for me. But food can be an emotional subject with people. Our society, for hundreds of years, has made food into a gift, a celebration, a reward, a show of respect, a sign of love, etc. Sometimes, when you turn down food being offered in this spirit, people are genuinely hurt and offended. And to those people I say: I'm sorry, but I just can't.

To me, food is none of those things and can never be again. It is just fuel for my life. That's all. So when I say "no thanks," don't take it personally.

FOOD IS NOT A REWARD

It starts out when we're young.

You do a good job in school, you behave when your parents need you to, you do a good job with your potty training.

And you're rewarded. Your parents give you candy. Or maybe a dessert. Maybe since you behaved during the time your parents shopped in the store, you're rewarded with a candy bar at the checkout stand. You make student of the month and your parents take you out for ice cream, or to your favorite fast-food restaurant.

We don't know it at the time, but these seemingly harmless, otherwise innocent acts are sowing the seeds for the weight problem that is rampaging throughout society today.

This is the habit that creates the association in our minds from a very young age: if I do something good, my body will receive food. Food is no longer a source of nourishment, a source of fuel for your body. It becomes a reward. Then what happens is this: as you get older in life, having had this reward system with food established, you begin to "treat" yourself.

You can see how this pattern continues for the rest of our lives. Do a good job at the office? Receive a pizza party. The company had a great quarter! Let's wheel in the junk food parade.

This is a disaster and it should stop, even though it never will. It's too ingrained in our psyche, but that doesn't mean we can't recognize it for what it is and seek to minimize it.

Well-meaning people have often asked me if I am going to celebrate weight-loss milestones by rewarding myself and eating something "special" or "a little extra." This is the exact cycle of behavior that got me into trouble in the first place, so why would I keep doing it?

So how do we stop the food-as-a-reward insanity? The solution is simple: just don't do it. There are other ways to reward people. How about money? Non-food gifts? A trip? Anything but food. Because as long as we as human beings believe food is a reward, we are going to strive to seek it out as much as possible and the weight struggle will continue forever.

It's time to break the association. Food is not entertainment. Food is not a celebration. Food is not a reward. Food is what we eat to survive. It is fuel for our bodies. Nothing more, nothing less.

STAY HUMBLE, MY FRIENDS

I recently saw a presentation where a woman was talking to her audience about how she had lost 400 pounds. What an amazing accomplishment. She did it all on her own, using basic common sense, just like I have. Only hers was more. I was blown away by her results.

And then I saw it. The cocky attitude. The arrogance. It became obvious to me watching her video that she believed she had the one and only true answer. If everyone wanting to lose weight would just do what she did, the world would be perfect. To hear her talk, you would think she was cured.

Only she's not. And neither am I, or anyone else. You see, my friends, that is the great lesson of weight loss. When you're losing weight, you have to realize that there is a very specific reason that greater than 9 out of 10 people who lose weight gain it all back.

It's hard. It's very, very, very hard. Nothing anyone has been doing, will be doing, has discovered or has yet to discover will change that.

I was once where she was. 15 years ago when I was losing all this weight once before, I was on top of the world. I thought I had all the answers. I would talk endlessly about my weight loss and how I was doing. How I had it all under control and no one else did. I thought I had found the secret. I had cracked the code. I was cured of my weight problem forever. I used to go around telling people "I'll never go back."

2 years later, I had fallen from that lofty perch straight back down into the deepest depths of my food addiction. I didn't just fall of the wagon....I dove head-first off of it at 100 miles an hour. I went from having an almost Zen-like ability to control everything I ate to eating non-stop, as much as I could, as fast as I could. Total control to zero control in 24 months.

Failure is a great teacher. I think about what I went through every day. And so I don't talk about my weight loss unless somebody brings it up. I don't offer my opinion about what anyone else is doing unless asked. I don't outwardly celebrate my weight loss. I do celebrate in private with people that are close to me, but that's it.

Why? Because I have to stay humble. I know what could happen. I know the deck is stacked. I know that I am only as good as my last workout. My last exercise. My last healthy meal. It will never end. The struggle will go on forever, only it will get harder. Temptation is always all around me. I'm very confident I have the right attitude this time, but I don't have all the answers. No one does.

I've said it before and I'll say it again: some days I feel like Superman. Other days, it is a struggle. On those days, I hate going to the gym. Some days I am hungry all the time and I have to take it one meal at a time. One snack at a time. I pound the water just to get through the day. It is a struggle. So if you're losing weight, just remember: there is no need to spike the ball.

The other day, a friend of mine pointed out another friend of mine who had recently gained a lot of weight.

"Look at them, they gained all that weight back."

I couldn't correct them fast enough: "It's very hard. That could be either one of us."

People see the results I've been able to achieve over the last 3 years and mistakenly assume that I am cured. I am not. I have not cracked the secret weight loss code, I have not found the Easy Button. I cannot sit here and say that I have lost this weight forever. Why?

Because we are all day-to-day. Back in 1999, I gained 250 pounds in about 9 months. It was the most humiliating experience of my life. That failure affects every decision I make today when it comes to managing this weight loss.

It's hard.

It's very, very hard. It can be done, but it is difficult. I am no better than anyone else. I have only figured out what works for me, for the moment. And really, it's just like any other addiction. But see, the thing about food addiction is you can't quit. You still have to eat. And you have to eat quite often.

But back to making fun of overweight people. Don't do it. It's rude, it's not nice and we go through enough condescension and humiliation in our lives, we don't need it from anyone else.

The high and mighty among us might look at the overweight person and cast aspersions on them. But what they don't realize is that one day, that very well might be them. They get older. Their metabolism slows down. They start eating more calories. Exercising less. Surprise, they've gotten heavy too.

I've said it before and I will say it again: the overweight are the last group of people it is acceptable to discriminate against. We know we're overweight, we don't need you to tell us. Being overweight, while ultimately the responsibility of the person that is heavy, is a creation of the American way of life in the 21st century.

So be nice. And if you're losing weight, stay humble.

PORTION DISTORTION

"Portion Distortion" is a great term used to describe how we perceive a large amount of food as a single serving. This will lead some people to say "I don't eat that much," when in fact, they're eating 5 servings. This could also be called denial, something I was an expert in, but that is another chapter.

Portion size is a huge issue for me. Obviously, having gotten my weight up to 577 pounds, I ate way too much. But how much is "too much?" How do you decide? Through my own experiences, I have come to the following conclusions about portion sizes:

I never trust my own eyes when it comes to portion sizes. I long ago came to the conclusion that my mind wants to keep me as heavy as possible. Sometimes, I will look at a plateful of food and think "that is a huge amount of food." Other times, I look at the *exact* same portion and think "that isn't very much."

That perception, what I think in my mind as being the appropriate amount of food, is never right. So I have learned not to trust it.

Measure, measure, measure. People who want to lose weight need to invest in 3 things: a measuring cup/spoon set, a food scale and a note pad. Measure and write it down. If you're trying to lose weight, never, ever, ever, ever trust your eye or mind when it comes to portion size. It cannot be trusted. You cannot guess. You cannot eat what looks "about right." To do so is to become a victim of Portion Distortion.

Use smaller plates. This seems simple, but I have found it very effective. Think about it: if you put your dinner on an 8" plate, it's going to look like a lot more food than if you put that same exact amount of food on a 12" plate. You will mindlessly fill your plate to capacity. Why should the size of the plate dictate how much you eat? That, my friends, is insanity.

Stay out of the restaurants. Portion Distortion is out of control at restaurants. The plates are huge. When you add up the chips/salsa, the bread, the appetizer, the soda, the salad, the entree, the dessert....restaurant meals are multiple thousands of calories. I believe it is next to impossible to lose weight and keep it off if you eat in restaurants all the time. I am sure it could be done, but I couldn't do it. Think about it: if somebody was going to give you everything you wanted without any limits, how are you going to keep track of it? That is what a restaurant is. Consider the endless refills of soda that are several hundred calories per serving.

Read labels. They're there, and people mostly ignore them. But look closely. How many servings are in the package you are eating out of? How on Earth do you eat an entire bag of chips that totals over 1,000 calories and fit that into a 2,400 calorie a day diet? You can't. Read the labels...it will open your eyes.

If you don't know how much you're eating, put it down and run away!

SETTLING AND DYING HAPPY

Losing weight and keeping it off is one of the hardest things there is to do in life. There's a very good reason many fail (like I have in the past) and really struggle with it (like I will for the rest of my life.)

So with the odds stacked so high against you, how do you succeed?

First, you have to find your motivation. Mine was simple: not dying. Staying alive. Yours might be to live a better life, to see your kids grow up, to be in shape, etc.

But I have another angle to consider. Set aside all of the common trains of thought about weight loss. Forget motivation, forget willpower. Forget discipline, forget diets. Forget it all and think about this:

Why should you accept being overweight? Why do you settle for that unhealthy lifestyle and all of the limitations that go with it? Especially if you're very overweight to the point of it limiting your mobility and inhibiting your social life like I was.

Don't settle. There is a better life everyone is capable of enjoying. I'm not sure if anyone is like me, but when I decide something is unacceptable, I draw a line in the sand and do something else.

"But I will just eat whatever I want and it makes me happy, so I will die happy."

That, my friends, is a lie. You won't die happy. This isn't Hollywood: "the big one" just doesn't painlessly take you out. Here's what really happens: you die a slow, miserable, death.

You get diabetes. You lose a limb. You have a stroke. You go blind. You're taking pill after pill after pill, constantly treating symptoms, but never the disease.

Your last years on this Earth are spent in the health care system. Constant doctor's visits. Endless trips to the ER. Non-stop medical attention and churning through the hospital. Mobility is restricted. Quality of life suffers.

All of that flashed before me when I was in the hospital 3 years ago and it lit a fire that burns inside me to this day. I only had to lay in that bed for about 2 days before I realized that the food wasn't worth it. It just isn't. Every food commercial will try to make you think it is, but it isn't.

If you have any weight to lose or if you just want to get back into shape and live a healthier life, don't wait. Don't wait until you're on the table in the ER wondering if you're done for.

Take action now. Throw away the soda and start drinking water. Stay out of the drive-thru. Go to the grocery store and buy some food instead of going to a restaurant. Make a healthy pizza with your family instead of ordering the garbage that gets delivered to your door.

PRIORITIES

"Remembering that you are going to die is the best way I know to avoid the trap of thinking you have something to lose."
-Steve Jobs, 2005

I started this chapter off with a quote from the late, great Steve Jobs because he can teach us all about living and dying. Several years before he lost his life to cancer, Steve Jobs gave a commencement address at Stanford University. It's only about 15 minutes long, but it is the best speech I have ever seen about life and death. Go to YouTube and type in "Steve Jobs commencement" and watch it. It is very inspirational and it is where that quote above comes from. (Go ahead, do it now and come back. I will be waiting.)

I've never been one to have clear-cut priorities in my life. I've always just done whatever I wanted to do, in whatever order I wanted to do it, whenever I felt like it. I've always envied people who had that single, driving passion from day 1 and followed it forever. That's just never been me.

I've also frequently put things (and people) ahead of myself. But like the Steve Jobs quote at the top of this posting says, nothing changes your perspective and priorities like realizing you are about to die. It does something to you. People used to tell me that, but I never understood what they were talking about until it happened to me.

3 years ago, on my way to the hospital, I was convinced I was having a heart attack and I was convinced I was about to die. For hours after that in the emergency room, I was still sure I was having heart problems and death was imminent. A cardiologist once told me they don't do open heart surgery on people over 500 pounds. So I was sure the grim reaper was knocking on the door and the game was over.

When I discovered I was going to live, but only with major changes in my life, it all became very clear. Like no other time in my first 37 years on this Earth, it all became crystal clear. I remember hearing myself say it over and over in my head laying in the hospital bed for 6 days straight:

"Nothing matters anymore except my health. Nothing."

And in one fell swoop, everything went out the window. All that mattered was my health. Doing what the doctors told me, following a regimen and setting up everything to support a healthy lifestyle was job #1. Anything that got in the way had to go. I am motivated by the will to live, no other reason.

For the first time in my life, I didn't care about anything else. I didn't care that I had wasted the first 37 years of my life being overweight. Who cares. All that mattered was I was alive. I remember looking up the average life expectancy in the United States on my Blackberry while I was in the hospital. (A Blackberry, I know. But hey, this was 2010. Give me a break. I have since upgraded.) According to the World Bank, it is 78 years.

So I did the math. I was 37 at the time. If I'm just average, that is 41 more years. What do I want those next 41 years to be like? Do I want to let my weight problem define me? Do I want to stay stuck in the past, squandering away the days, weeks, months and years by worrying about the past?

The answer is and remains NO. The battle cry became NO MORE. I would get so worked up in the hospital, I would pound my fists on the tray table over my bed and shout "NO MORE!." The nurses must have thought I had gone insane. But I had had enough. No more.

From that point forward, everything else ceased to matter. I no longer cared:

-What other people thought about me
-About my career
-How I looked
-What I wore
-If people talked about me
-How much money I made or didn't make
-What anyone else did or didn't do

All that mattered was staying alive. Like Steve Jobs says in that commencement video, death has a way of doing that to you. You realize what matters. Everything else washes away. None of it matters.

So what motivates me? The will to live. I'm not done with my life yet. I want more. This needs to be you.

WHY NOT JUST STOP?

I used to get the question all the time when I weighed over 500 pounds.

"Why not just stop eating so much?"

The answer to that ridiculous question is not easy. But the simple answer is this: because you can't. It's like any other addiction. Why doesn't the drug addict stop doing cocaine? Why don't you stop smoking? Why don't you stop drinking coffee? Why don't you stop drinking alcohol? Why don't you stop eating fast food? And on and on.

The more I think about it and the longer my lifestyle change goes on (3 years and counting,) the more I realize there is no sure-fire, guaranteed way for anyone to change their life permanently before they're ready.

You can give someone the information.

You can be supportive.

You can show them the way.

But there is no way you can do it for them.

But I know what doesn't work. Diets. Gimmicks. Fads. Living off frozen dinners. Starvation. None of it works. Sure, you'll lose weight. But what do those plans offer you 5 years out? Right. Nothing.

So how does someone change?

They change because they (not you, not me, not anything or anyone else) reach a point where they can't take it anymore. But they have to arrive at this point. There is nothing you can say to them to get them to change.

Nothing, nothing, nothing.

No one could tell me anything to make me change my lifestyle before I hit rock bottom and almost died. There was not a thing in the world anyone could do or say. It was only when I decided to make it all happen that it was going to happen. The same goes for you.

And one final thing: if somebody has lost a bunch of weight in the past and then gained it all back, please do not say "You did it before, you can do it again. You know what works!" to them. If they gained all the weight back, their plan failed. It didn't work. Repeating it over again is only going to achieve the same results.

RAGE AGAINST THE WEIGHT LOSS MACHINE

It's the million dollar question: how do you get motivated to lose weight? I get asked it all the time. I will tell you where mine comes from:

Anger.

That's right. Anger. Rage. But at who? At what? For what reason?

You can be mad at yourself for allowing yourself to get to your current state (whatever that is.)

Or, you can do what I do, which is to get mad at the entire food and weight-loss industry. All of it.

First on my list: restaurants, specifically fast-food chains. I hate them all. You run food commercials on TV, making it unwatchable for food addicts like me. You put photographs of your garbage food on billboards and litter the landscape pushing your drug. Actually, we all know nothing you sell looks like the food in the billboards or the commercials, that's just part of the deception. There is nothing of any positive nutritional value in a fast-food restaurant and if there is, it is only there to lure people in and make them feel alright about eating there.

Not fired up enough yet? Let's move on to the food companies.

The US government requires that pet food be solely nutritious enough to sustain the animal it is being fed to. In other words, the government has higher standards for dog food than it does for the garbage being pumped out by the food companies.

You load your "food" up with so much fat, sugar and salt and put it in a box with a pretty picture on the front. You peddle your garbage to kids. The processed food industry poisons the population with its trash with reckless abandon. The final insult? We pay for it all. The US government subsidizes crops like corn, which is used to make trash like high fructose corn syrup so cheaply that the food companies use it over more healthy ingredients.

It's well-known that food companies play games with the serving size on labels to make their food look better nutritionally than what it is. Some of the serving sizes are ridiculously small, like a major soda company claiming 2.5 servings in a 20 ounce bottle of soda.

Or take bread. Serving size: 1 slice. Who eats 1 slice of bread? Nobody. You make a sandwich, so really, 1 serving is 2 slices. I could go on, but you get the idea.

The food companies are afraid that people will find out what is *really* in their food. That's why they make 1 can of soup have 2 servings in it, because if you really knew it contained almost 2,000mg of sodium, you might run the other way.

And last, but certainly not least, my favorite target: the weight-loss industry.

Let me be clear: the weight-loss industry is a criminal cartel of companies whose executives should be arrested, companies shut down and the money stolen from its victims given back.

I'm talking about them all. The pills. The surgeries. The frozen dinners. The diet books. The broken promises. The lies. The scams. The phony claims about results almost no one gets.

These thieves should be locked up. But for some reason, they are allowed to continue to rip people off. It is a 100% truth that the weight-loss industry is the only industry that sells a product that when it doesn't work, the consumer blames themselves. No responsibility is ever shared by the company that created the rip-off product that doesn't work.

There are many rip-offs and deceptions in our society, but there is none greater than that which is perpetrated on the American people by the weight loss industry.

No other crooked enterprise even comes close. The guys running the Nigerian money transfer scam can only dream of ripping people off on such a grand scale. Used car salesmen look like fine, upstanding members of society compared to the weight loss companies. But here's why it works. Here's why the con is so perfect.

People are so desperate for a quick fix, they're so desperate for the easy way out, they are willing to believe anything. And my friends when I say anything, I do mean anything.

You see the commercials. You see a famous football player on TV telling you how much weight he lost and how great he feels. You see the ripped muscle guy on TV using some stupid machine you can buy for 4 payments of $99.99 and you think...hey, that could be me! (Only it won't be you, ever.)

You know who I'm talking about: the diets, the infomercials, the books, the pills, the machines, etc.

Do people really think there is such a thing as a "fat-burning" pill? It is amazing that something with such a high failure rate continues to make its inventors so rich.

What sucks so much about this whole thing is not only are people's money being stolen by these thieves, their hope is being taken away. People who are suffering in an overweight prison and feel so desperate for something....anything...to help them lose weight buy this trash.

Then, when it doesn't work (it never was going to work in the first place,) they give up.

That is a tragedy. If any other industry released a product with a 90%+ failure rate, the product would be taken off the market, the company sued out of existence and their owners arrested and put in jail.

But no, not the weight-loss industry. They get a pass. There's millions to be made because there's a sucker born every minute, desperately looking for the easy way out.

But here is the 100% truth: none of it works. None of it was ever going to work, all of it is guaranteed to fail 100% of the time. Oh, you'll lose weight. Lots of people lose weight. There will be success stories. That's how they get into the ads.

But think about it, be honest with yourself. Are you really going to order frozen dinners off the television and eat them the rest of your life? No.

Are you really going to shake a weight in your hand every day and achieve dreams of muscle-bound glory? No.

Are you really going to only eat meat for the rest of your life, swearing off carbohydrates forever? Nope.

If you can't do it for the rest of your life, it isn't worth doing. Losing a whole bunch of weight that you can't keep off is an enormous waste of time. I know, I was there once. I lost 240 pounds 13 years ago using an extreme diet and exercise plan I could not keep up and guess what? I gained it all back, plus 137 more pounds. It was a traumatic failure.

And here is what is all the more amazing: a diet is the only product where people blame themselves when it doesn't work. Imagine buying a television, taking it home and having it die after a week. You wouldn't say "Oh, I must've done something wrong. I wasn't doing it right." No, you would put it back in the box, march it back to the store and demand a refund. Only when it comes to the diets and the weight loss rip-offs, people don't do that. Incredible.

So, to recap:

1.) All diets are doomed to fail as a means of long-term weight loss.

2.) There is no magic pill, machine or special food that is going to make you lose weight.

3.) There is no such thing as a "fat burner." You are the only possible fat burner yourself, when you move your body and exercise.

4.) The best diet plan is one that you create and customize yourself, using common sense.

Don't be ripped off, my friends. Keep your money and spend it at the grocery store.

That should give you an idea of where I am coming from.

One final note: being angry at somebody or something and using it for motivation is not the same as blaming them. I and I alone am responsible for my weight problem. I put the food in my mouth and eat it, no one else.

Past that, they can all go to hell. Now get to work!

RESTAURANT ADDICTION

Of all the things I have changed in my life in the last 3 years, nothing causes more controversy than my "no restaurants" pledge.

It really bothers people. I don't know why. Perhaps because I am so inflexible. Perhaps because eating out in restaurants is such a fabric of our lives, such a part of the American way of life in the 21st century. Eating in restaurants is a way to socialize, a way to celebrate. We do it all the time without thinking and can't imagine not doing it. Being served by someone else in a fancy restaurant is a status symbol, a sign of success.

But I'm not going to do it and here's why.

I've said over and over that I am a food addict. It's my problem. For the first 37 years of my life, I abused food. I still do sometimes and have to be careful.

If food was my drug then the restaurant was my crack house.

What is the purpose of a restaurant? Why is it there? Like any other business, its sole purpose is to make money. And there is nothing wrong with that. We live in a capitalistic society and the restaurant owner has every right to operate their business as they see fit.

But the restaurant owner does not care about:

-Serving you anything remotely healthy
-The quality of the food (only the taste)
-Limiting your intake. On the contrary, they want you to eat as much as possible

The restaurant owner also has to keep an eye on food costs. Since the goal is to get you to spend as much as possible, that means serving you as much food, as cheaply as possible that tastes as good as possible. And for most people, tasting good means as much sugar, salt and fat as possible.

None of those are good for me. It's a bad environment for a food addict. Something happens to me when the consumption of food is turned into an entertainment occasion. When everyone is laughing and having a good time and the server is bringing me anything I want, as much as I want...self-control melts away. Who keeps track in a restaurant? Hardly anyone.

So like an alcoholic does not belong in a bar, I do not belong in a restaurant. I do not begrudge anyone their restaurant experience. I'm the one with the problem.

They're just not for me.

So what about you? Am I telling you to never eat in a restaurant ever again, as long as you live? That is what I have done and it has worked for me. It forces you to manage your own nutrition. Since everything you eat comes from the grocery store and is managed by you, you maintain total control.

I can hear it now, but Bryan...what about special occasions? Graduations? Weddings? Business luncheons and dinners I cannot get out of? It turns out I have some experience in this area. A few years ago, I had a business dinner I couldn't get out of. I had to go. Thankfully, it was at a 5-star restaurant and the server got with the chef and made a healthy dinner that met my requirements. That was the first, only and last time I have dined out during my 3-year lifestyle change.

In other words, it was RARE. You see, that's how restaurants used to be in our society. Going out to eat used to be a special occasion. Once in awhile. NOT every day. Or every week. Or every month. Mom made dinner and society didn't have the weight problem it does.

So I have developed a guide to dining out. Are you ready for it? Here goes:

YOU ARE ALLOWED TO EAT OUT 4 TIMES A YEAR. NO MORE.

What?!?!? Only 4 times a year? That's impossible! I'll dry up and blow away! I'll have to tell people "no." I'm used to getting everything I want! I won't survive.

No, it is perfect. 4 times a year about covers your "special occasion" needs. That's enough for a wedding, a graduation, a Thanksgiving or a business dinner or luncheon you can't get out of. 4 times, no more.

If you do not put yourself in charge of what you eat and how much you eat, your lifestyle change will never take hold. Remember: the restaurant owner's goal is to get you to eat as much as possible. You are not a dog. You do not just eat what your master puts in a bowl.

Apply that logic to other areas of your life. Just as the restaurant decides your portion size and the contents of your food, what if your boss dictated to you how much you would be paid? What if you had no say? Same thing. You have to maintain control.

Normal people can eat in a restaurant and not overeat. But our dirty little secret is we are not normal people. You've got to find a way to stay out of the restaurants.

You have to be the captain of your own nutritional ship.

Over the course of my 3-year weight loss journey, I have heard from a lot of people.

People who saw my story on CNN or watched my video on YouTube will e-mail me asking for advice. They want to know how to get my results. A lot of people are really struggling with weight issues.

But when I drill down into their lifestyle and eating habits, I find a very familiar common thread:

People cannot stay out of the restaurants.

Whether it's the instant gratification, the ability to have anything you want at anytime or just the convenience, people love the drive-thrus and the delivery drivers. They love restaurants. There is only one problem.

You are killing yourself at the restaurants. Sure, we ultimately pull the trigger…but the restaurant loads the gun.

For someone who has a weight problem, everything about a restaurant feeds into an out-of-control lifestyle. The gigantic portions, the free refills.....the buffets. It is all a recipe for disaster. People will sit and consume 1,000 calories of breadsticks before the entree even arrives.

And the worst part about restaurants? It makes us lazy. Somebody else is deciding everything for us. We have zero input into what we're eating and how much we're eating. The restaurant decides the portion.

If you make it yourself, you know what's in it. You know how much you're eating. You're cooking a meal as your own chef, not as a salesman trying to boost your final bill as much as possible.

OK, so let's face a few facts about the food that's widely available. Vending machine "food." Restaurant food. A lot of grocery store food. Food on television commercials. Food prepared on the TV food shows.

The food sucks. And it sucks bad.

If it's high in sodium, your food sucks. I have not busted my hump for 3 years and slowly worked my way off of several medications just so I can eat something that has thousands of milligrams of sodium in it.

If your food is super-high in fat, it sucks. And I am not a fat Nazi. There is such a thing as healthy fats. There is such a thing as reasonableness. But really? Some of these fast food meals are OUTRAGEOUS. It's not food, it's slow-acting poison.

Or how about the food in the vending machines. 600 calories for a honey bun? Are you serious? That's as many calories as in my entire breakfast. And I get a bowl of oatmeal, a banana, scrambled egg whites. Sausage patties. What are you eating? Garbage.

And delivery pizzas? More slow-acting poison. It all sucks.

It's not so much that the food is bad for you or that it is high in fat, calories and sodium...it's just that YOUR FOOD SUCKS.

The quality is bad. You're not getting anything in return for the hit on your waistline. The food just sucks.

There is better food to be had, but you're going to have to make it yourself. At least you'll know what you put in it.

MAKE YOUR BUCKET LIST

When I was in the hospital 3 years ago with a lot of time to kill on my hands, I made a "Bucket List" of sorts. It was exactly what it says: things I wanted to be able to do once I lost weight, before I "kicked the bucket."

I wrote down on a legal pad all of the things my extra weight was preventing me from doing. As you can imagine, at 577 pounds my mobility was really suffering. So here are some of the things I wanted to be able to do, that I couldn't at that time:

Sit in any chair. That's right, I would go to the doctor's office and I couldn't sit down. Why? All of the chairs had arms and they were too close together for me to sit in them. I can now sit in any chair I want at any time. And cross my legs. How about that!

Fly in an airplane. I got to do this a couple years ago when my company flew me to New Jersey on business. First time I had been in an airplane in 12 years and it was a fantastic feeling. I have since flown across the country on a small plane, in coach no less.

Buy clothes at the regular store. When I was in the hospital, I was too big to buy clothes even at the big and tall store. I dreamed of buying clothes at the regular store. Regular sizes for regular prices, just like a regular person. I now buy my clothes at any store I want and haven't been to the big and tall store in over a year

Find the smallest rental car I can and drive it. This item was on the list because in recent years, I had wanted to take a trip, but couldn't because I wouldn't fit in any of the cars for rent. I have since driven some of the smallest cars you can imagine, with plenty of room.

Get a bicycle and ride it. I had always dreamed of riding a bicycle again. I had gotten too big to ride my bicycle years ago and always wanted to do it again. I have been riding a ten speed bicycle a friend gave me and it is liberating. I'm up to over 26 miles at a time.

Enter the local "Cooper River Bridge Run" 10K race. Ever since I moved to Charleston, SC in 2005, I had always seen this event going on and dreamed that one day I would be able to participate. I am proud to report that in the last 3 years, I have participated in the race 3 times in a row. Even as I am typing these words, I can't believe it. This is like a fantasy come true.

To be able to fit in all of the test equipment and machines at the hospital. This one was on the list because while I was in the hospital, they couldn't do a CT scan on me. The weight limit for that machine is something like 360 pounds and at 577 pounds, it was no go. Not too long ago, I went for a routine CT scan of my lungs and I fit right in the machine. If radiation exposure weren't a concern, I would go back and have one done ever few months, just because I can.

To be able to have blood drawn easily. I have said over and over again in this book as well as in person that when it comes to the benefits of my weight loss, it is the little things that matter most.

For almost my entire lifetime, because of my weight, whenever I would go have blood drawn, it would be an absolute never-ending disaster. Lab tech after lab tech, nurse after nurse and sometimes doctors would try to find a vein from which to draw blood. It was a huge production and they would almost always all fail.

I have been stuck up to 10 times just to get one vial of blood. I have had it taken out of my fingers, my hands, my arms, my wrists and just about everywhere else except for my eyeball. I have had multiple tourniquets on my arm wrapped so tightly I thought my arm was going to pinch off and fall to the floor.

What's worse, because I was on blood thinners for a long time due to my pulmonary embolism 3 years ago, I had to have blood drawn once a month to be sure it is not clotting and that I am on the right amount of Coumadin.

But my friends, no more.

Recently, for the third time in a row, all 3 tubes of blood were drawn with a single stick, right in my arm, just like everybody else.

There were no multiple sticks. There were no multiple tries. There were no nurses "going to get the doctor." I was in and out in under 3 minutes. You want motivation to lose weight? It's the little things.

So there you have it. A sample from my Bucket List, 3 years ago today. What's on your bucket list? Go ahead and make one. What are some of the things you have always wanted to do, but can't? Are you tired of not being able to keep up with your kids? If so, WRITE IT DOWN. Your life is waiting…make it happen!

THE WRONG IDEA ABOUT EATING

A lot of people have the wrong idea (and so did I) that they are overweight solely because they eat too much.

This brings along with it the following baggage:

1.) Emotions of guilt and shame over eating

2.) Becoming overly conscious of what people think about your eating habits

3.) Feeling like you're being judged all the time

The truth is, you have to eat. Every last person on this Earth must eat food daily or you will eventually die. I would argue the overweight person (myself included, 3 years ago) is overweight because they aren't eating enough food, aren't eating it at the right time and are eating the wrong things.

In other words, there's no plan.

And another thing. Society is so cruel to overweight people. We are not victims by any stretch, we do eat the food that makes us overweight. But we are also vastly growing in numbers as a side effect of the American way of life.

So back to the title of this chapter: "the wrong idea about eating."

I eat more now in volume than I did when I weighed 577 pounds. But it is WHAT I am eating that makes my body weight so much different. I am not "eating too much," I am eating the right amount.

One last point: no one, no matter how successful they have or have not been at weight loss should stand in judgment of anyone else. People ask me to do this all the time. "Look at that person. They should do what you did."

We are all day to day. I am no better than anyone else. I have lost large amounts of weight before (although not this much) and gained it all back. Had I not almost died from multiple blood clots in my lungs 3 years ago, I would probably weigh 650 pounds by now.

You have to eat. You should be eating quite a lot to nourish your body. There is nothing wrong or bad about eating. Food is life!

WHAT DO I EAT? YES, THERE ARE BAD FOODS

I get asked all the time:

"Are cereal bars OK?"

"Can I eat this or that?"

"What about fat-free this, or light that?"

Here's the problem. All of those may be perfectly fine, but you're barking up the wrong tree. Read the next sentence and commit it to memory:

You need to eat food that will fill you up.

Starving yourself, eating diet food, eating ridiculously small portions, eating frozen dinners...it's all a short-term recipe for failure. Sure, your calories will be restricted and you will lose weight, but you're not going to be able to keep it up.

A better idea is to eat healthy food in abundance. Eat until you are full, until you don't want anymore. I call it the 6 food groups:

1.) **Fruits.** Find fruits you like and eat them all.

2.) **Vegetables.** Same thing. Find ones you like and eat them.

3.) **Lean meats and beans.** Baked fish. Baked chicken breast. Grilled. Pork. Turkey. All kinds of beans. Cook your own or do what I do: get the "no salt added" kind that come in a box or a can.

4.) **Whole grains.** Really heavy, high-fiber wheat bread. Brown rice. Oatmeal.

5.) **Low fat dairy.** Fat-free milk. Non fat yogurt, etc.

6.) **Water.** (yes, with my plan, water is a food group.) At least a gallon a day.

You are *not* going to be successful, long-term, for the rest of your life, eating tiny portions, energy bars, cereal bars or diet food.

Eat real food! And eat a lot! Stay full!

You've heard it before:

"There are no bad foods."

"You can eat anything in moderation."

Now, these two statements might be true for you. Everyone is different. If you only have 10 or 20 pounds to lose or are just a little out of shape, maybe you really can eat anything in moderation.

But for those of us who are or were 100 or more pounds overweight, "anything" is not moderation. And yes, there are bad foods. Very,

very, very bad foods.

As a food addict (an actual real addiction with life-threatening consequences, not a jokey, made-up condition,) I absolutely cannot eat certain things. If I were to buy a bag of Doritos and eat them, putting that garbage in my mouth would cause 2 disasters.

One, it would undo in one fell swoop 3 years of work in modifying my taste buds. Over a long period of time, I have been able to rework my palate into not needing highly stimulating levels of fat, sugar and salt to feel satisfied.

Second, it would trigger a completely out of control binge. I wouldn't be able to stop. All of the bad habits, destructive behaviors and dangerous lifestyle would come flooding back. It would be the start of a slow suicide and a descent back into the hell of being hundreds of pounds overweight. Yes, that's right, all of that would happen eating a single bag of Doritos. Sorry to be so dramatic, but it's true.

Some people can eat the garbage food like a squirrel. A little bit here and there, most of it tucked away to eat later. I am not some people. I cannot touch the stuff. It is like radioactive poison to me.

But increasingly, more and more people, myself included, need to realize they must stay away from it forever. It's not food. It's garbage. And it's going to kill you.

So yes, there are bad foods. What do you do? Walk away. This is the hardest thing to do and one of the biggest reasons sustained weight maintenance is so hard. We temporarily change our behaviors to experience short-term weight loss, only to return to them later. This is when the weight comes back.

I don't have a good answer for how to prevent that. But I do know this: what has worked for me has been simply abstaining from eating the trash that comes to us from fast-food restaurants, vending machines and pizza delivery drivers (sorry guys.)

Candy? Garbage. Fast food? It's trash. It's not "food" anyway, it's a science experiment. Cookies? More garbage. But the cookies are for a good cause and support my daughter's troop! Sorry, especially worthless garbage. Junk food is slow-acting poison that is going to kill us all.

I believe that if you switch to eating healthy food and continue to shop at the grocery store, your palate will adjust and you won't want the trash anymore.

And lastly, know this: food is absolutely used as a drug. The food companies and restaurant chains use fat, sugar and salt to hook you on the garbage. There is a reason you can't eat just one. It's because the substance has been manufactured to make it impossible to eat just one.

So don't do it. Walk away. Your life will be longer because you did.

WHEN YOU STRUGGLE (AND YOU WILL)

As anyone who has decided to make a lifestyle change knows, there are going to be struggles.

Struggling can take many forms. Suddenly, everything is harder than it used to be. You've gotten out of your routine. You've gotten lax on the food journaling and have quit keeping track. You haven't been going to the gym.

Then the panic sets in. Ridiculous thoughts race through your head: "Have all the old habits come back? Am I going to gain all the weight back? Am I not able to do it anymore? Were all my critics right? Am I doomed?"

No.

As someone who has failed spectacularly in the past, I at least have a little authority on the subject and I use that experience to help myself.

The great thing about the human body is it is the most advanced machine on the face of the Earth. No matter what has happened, no matter what you have or haven't done, you can always press the "reset" button.

You can always begin anew. Because it's not about losing weight. It's all about maintaining a healthy lifestyle. And when it gets hard, and I promise it will, you don't need to panic.

You just need a plan.

If you're in the beginning stages of your journey, where everything is coming easy and you feel indestructible, put some thought into what you'll do when it gets hard.

I'll use my own example.

Last year was not kind to me health-wise. I had strep throat, a sinus infection, a cold that wouldn't go away and then another sinus infection. I missed quite a bit of work and quite a bit of my gym routine.

What this did was upset the applecart. My routine had been interrupted. Some days all I felt like doing was eating. The old demons started to come back. But I know from experience that all I had to do was get through the day. Tomorrow is a new day, a different day. Everything will be different.

Nothing bad has happened. I have continued to lose weight. So now I am mixing it up, as my health improves. I am buying some new music. Hitting the gym again. Starting a new running routine. I just have to engage my mind and get back on the horse, but in a different way. Nothing is forever. What has worked for the first 3 years of my journey might need to change.

As for the idea that you can fall off the wagon once and somehow gain all the weight back right away, that is really nonsense and is physically impossible. The nearly 400 pounds I have lost, at 3,500 calories per pound, totals 1,400,000 calories. That means I would have to eat over 1 million calories in one sitting to gain all the weight back.

That's a lot of oatmeal and bananas.

WORKOUT MUSIC

When you undergo a total lifestyle change, you quickly learn that sometimes it's the little things that get you through the day.

For example, when it comes to working out. Whether you're walking, running or working out on a machine, the music you select is very, very important.

After doing this for 3 years, allow me to dispense a little advice. The music you should be working out to isn't necessarily going to be the music you like. It needs to be:

-Upbeat. You're not going to be working out to acoustic folk music or classical music. I suppose you could try, but I don't see Mozart pushing me to the limit.

-Motivational. Cue the "Rocky" music.

-Transformational. That is, the music should take you to another place.

-Imaginative. The music should make you imagine your goals, imagine yourself achieving them. Imagine the reaction of the naysayers. Visualize your success.

-Emotional. The music should push you...it should remind you of all that you have accomplished or want to accomplish.

I cannot stress the importance of the music having a very good beat. Because if it has a good, driving, pounding beat, the faster the beat, the faster you will go. So having read that, you can see why the music you like isn't necessarily the music you want to work out to. For instance, if you're a big fan of James Taylor or Dan Fogelberg....that just won't sustain you on an intense workout.

I listen to pounding, driving dance music. I also look for only upbeat music that is currently in the top 40. For some reason, new music helps me "stay young" in my mind and forces me to work out harder in the gym. Find out what motivates you and implement it.

I also put things on my iPhone like the Rocky theme. Because when I am gutting it out on the treadmill and I hear that music....with sweat pouring off my face....for a moment, I believe I am Rocky Balboa. I'm training for the next big fight. If "Eye of the Tiger" gets you amped up, listen to it. I know one person that listens exclusively to explicit rap music when he works out. At no other time in his life does he listen to this music, but it makes him push himself in the gym.

Again, it's the little things. Select your workout music based on how it makes you feel and how you will perform while listening to it.

THE GREAT CLOTHES LINE

Many people have advanced to me the idea that they are going to get into shape or lose weight and they will do this by purchasing a treadmill. The thinking goes that they will do this because:

1.) They can work out in the privacy of their own home. They don't have to worry about other people in the gym staring at them and judging their appearance.

2.) It will "just be there" to use anytime they need it, so that means they'll work out more.

3.) They will save on a gym membership because they will own their own equipment.

What a great idea! Well, except....allow me to inject a little reality into the treadmill-purchasing dreams of others with a new list:

1.) Your $500 treadmill (or $1,000...or whatever you spend) will make a great clothes-dryer.

2.) Because it is always available, you will never use it. If you can do it anytime you want, that makes it ripe for procrastination. Imagine if you had a homework assignment with no due date...would you ever do it? Nope.

3.) Unless you drop multiple thousands of dollars, the home version treadmills are nothing like the ones at the gym. They break easily and will need to be serviced. So much for the savings.

The reason I always took off like a rocket at the beginning of the year, but then fizzled with my New Year's resolutions to lose weight was because there was no accountability. There was no follow-through. Like a lot of people, instead of starting off slowly, I would overdo it. Then I would give up because I injured myself or thought I had to maintain a ridiculous training schedule of working out 20 times a week.

The whole reason for having a personal trainer is accountability. The reason I make an appointment then actually follow through with it is because I know that person is there waiting for me to come to the gym. If you don't have access to a personal trainer or can't afford one, find an accountability partner. And make it somebody that will actually hold you accountable, somebody you know that already works out.

Also, slow down. Slow way down. Don't expect to go from doing no exercise to being an Olympic athlete in 2 days. Try walking 3 times a week around your neighborhood for 15 or 30 minutes. Then maybe incorporate 2 gym visits a week.

And save that treadmill cash for something else...like treating yourself to a new wardrobe when you lose 30 pounds after following the advice above.

FAILURE IS A GIFT

"Success consists of going from failure to failure without loss of enthusiasm." -Winston Churchill

You may remember from earlier in this book that I once lost all of this weight back in 1997 and 1998.

And then I gained all of it back, plus more. It was complete and total epic failure on an absolutely cosmic scale. It was humiliating and painful.

That failure haunted me for over a decade. But when I was going through the weight loss, I felt indestructible. I felt like I had cracked the code and was cured forever. I was wrong.

So, when it all came crashing down, I panicked. Instead of just calmly trying something else and giving myself a break, I overreacted. It took me less than a year to gain back what I worked so hard for almost 2 years to lose. I have never been more humbled in my life.

When I set out to lose this weight again, I decided to learn as much as I could from my failure 12 years ago. Why didn't my plan work? Looking back now, I can see all the dumb things I was doing that were unsustainable:

1.) **I was starving myself.** Losing weight became the focus, rather than focusing on maintaining a healthy weight. I got addicted to the number on the scale. With that in mind, I only weigh on the scale every 2 weeks. Not 1 day sooner.

2.) **The foods I were eating were a drastic departure from a normal diet.** I became a vegetarian and for a time, a vegan. Those are healthy diets and good choices for some people, but unsustainable for me. This time I have tried to eat only the way that I think I can maintain forever.

3.) **I never cut myself a break**. When I gained back 5 or 10 pounds, I should've just relaxed and slowly gotten back on the horse. Back then, if i didn't go to the gym 10 times a week, I felt like a failure. I had completely lost my mind and it's no wonder I burned out. So these days I try and take the long view. If I miss a workout, I just go the next day and move on.

It really is true when people say "slow and steady wins the race." I'm not trying to win an award, just get and stay healthy.

The important thing is never giving up.

ONE MORE TIME, THERE IS NO SECRET

At first it's funny, but now it's just sad. If I had a nickel for every time somebody asked me "what the secret was," I would have enough to pay off the national debt.

I hate to burst anyone's bubble, but when it comes to sustained weight loss, there is no secret. It's long, it's hard, it's a lot of work. Sometimes I don't want to do the exercise. I don't want to eat breakfast every day. I'm not even hungry in the morning. But I make myself eat, so I don't get hungry later on.

People, it's hard. So let's forget about these popular theories:

1.) "I will lose weight when I find something that works." Sorry, the only thing that makes you lose weight is taking in less energy than you put out. It's an earth-shattering concept that works every time it is applied.

2.) Stop with the gimmicks, or at least stop telling me about them. There is no pill, plan, diet, machine, DVD, gym you can join then never go to, or any of it that is going to lose weight for you.

3.) Please stop telling me you "don't eat that much." I told myself that for decades and it never did any good. Yes, it's true. If I was hundreds of pounds overweight, I really did eat that much.

4.) You can't eat "anything in moderation" because anything is not moderation. Come on.

5.) And for crying out loud, please don't tell me how difficult it all is while at the same time stuffing your face with the contents of a fast food bag. (You know who you are...I still love you, but c'mon.)

No one has the answer for you, only you do. No one else is going to fix your life. It has to come from within.

So from now on, when people ask me my secret, I'm going to tell them I did it all with that weight you shake in your hand (just kidding.)

Oh, and one more thing: the weight-loss patch only works if you put it over your mouth.

As near as I can tell, here are the "secrets:"

Motivation. You either have this or you don't. You either want to lose weight, or you don't. That's something that comes from within, you can't make yourself lose weight. You have to want to do it.

Avoid getting hungry and eat early and often. I eat 6 meals a day and about 2,400 calories a day. That's actually a fair amount of food. If you portion your food, measure it and keep a food diary, you will be able to eat all day.

Eat breakfast. A nurse in the hospital told me that all the heavy people she knew didn't eat breakfast. When you don't eat breakfast, you start out the day starving. Bad idea. The hunger builds throughout the day and by the nighttime, you've not eaten much all day and start binging. At least that's what I used to do.

Pay attention to what you eat and what's in it. You can really eat anything....you just have to realize what you're eating.

Don't go to extremes. Don't starve yourself. Don't work out like a maniac. All you're doing is setting yourself up for failure. You can't push a button and drop 100 pounds. However, if you do have a button like that, send me an e-mail.

Weight is lost at the dinner table more than it is in the gym. Exercise has a poor rate of return when it comes to weight loss. You can erase an entire workout with one trip through the drive-thru. The point is, it is impossible to out-exercise a diet of bad choices.

So there you have it: my weight loss secrets. Boring, huh? Sorry.

WHY NOT HAVE WEIGHT LOSS SURGERY?

Why not have weight loss surgery?

I often get the question asking me why I didn't or don't have weight loss surgery. It's a simple question with a complex answer.

First of all, I don't judge people that have had weight loss surgery. For many people, that is their last option. And many people do have tremendous success and results with the surgery (at least at first.)

Why didn't I have the surgery? I could have. I've worked 3 places in the last 10 years that would've paid for the surgery in full. The reason I never did it was because I always knew that I could do it myself if I just put out the effort.

I also knew that if I wasn't committed to losing weight the regular way, I wouldn't be committed to it with the gastric bypass.

After I wound up in the hospital with the pulmonary embolism 3 years ago, I got very tired of being in the hospital. That was one long week. So, I decided before I went with the gastric bypass, I would try one last time.

That was 3 years ago.

But I take nothing away from people that have the gastric bypass surgery. There are risks, complications and it is a lot of long, hard work to lose weight. They are doing what's right for them. If the result is a longer, healthier, happier life, then how you got there doesn't matter.

Being overweight is being on the wrong end of a math problem. More energy is being consumed than is being expended. Whatever you have to do to restore that balance is key.

I believe weight loss surgery should be restored to what it originally was, an option of last resort for somebody who is absolutely immobile and is hopelessly overweight to the point that they are going to die if they don't do something soon.

But that's just me giving my opinion (you can do that when you write a book.)

THE 7 HABITS OF HEALTHY PEOPLE

It's become obvious to me that there are certain behaviors and certain things that healthy people do that we could all stand to follow. Some of these I do, some of them I should do more of.

So with apologies to the late, great Stephen Covey, I present to you the 7 habits of healthy people:

1.) **Healthy people eat all the time.** It's true, I've seen it in action...and now I do it. Healthy people realize that the body is a machine and the machine needs fuel. You can't treat your body like a car, driving around on E all the time and only filling up at the last possible minute. If you don't eat often, then you become very hungry and desperate, which leads to poor decision-making and binge eating on unhealthy foods.

2.) **Healthy people are prepared.** You have to eat every day, several times a day...day in and day out, week in and week out. Healthy people stock up and have food on hand. My health and wellness coach at the gym I go to sits at his desk eating peanut butter out of the jar with a banana. He wouldn't dream of not packing his lunch and neither would I. The food has to come from somewhere and healthy people don't get it from vending machines, the drive-thru or the pizza delivery guy.

3.) **Healthy people don't kill themselves in the gym.** The people I know who stay in shape do not work out 4 hours a day in the gym 10 times a week. They have a regular schedule where they go 3 or 4 times a week, about an hour a day. Nothing crazy. This allows the healthy person to maintain a healthy weight, stay in shape and not burn out.

4.) **Healthy people work exercise into their daily routine.** Whether it's taking the stairs, parking far away from the store entrance, going for a walk or something else, healthy people integrate physical activity into their daily lives somehow. That way, "working out" is not the only source of physical activity. The healthy person does not drive around the mega mart parking lot for 20 minutes waiting for the magic parking spot by the front door to open (which I used to do.)

5.) **Healthy people keep it simple.** I love technology. But in my observations, most healthy people I know don't scan bar codes into their phones at the grocery store or walk around with a tracker all day long adding up their movements. You don't need a special machine to work out and you don't need a smart phone app to track how much you eat. I use a pen and paper.

6.) **Healthy people don't avoid the doctor.** I did it for years. I would never go to the doctor until the last possible minute. I was always flirting with disaster and my stupidity almost cost me my life. Healthy people go to the doctor, get checked out, get treated for any problems and keep it moving.

7.) **Healthy people grocery shop a lot.** Every healthy person I know, whether it be a personal trainer, a running enthusiast or a body builder...they load up at the grocery store once in awhile. The healthy person realizes that there is nothing healthier than the food they prepare themselves, because they know what's in it. Since healthy people get most of their food from the grocery store, dining out becomes the exception rather than the rule.

If you want to be a healthy person, do what healthy people do. Those 7 things should get you started. Now go....go do it now!

WALKING IS THE EXERCISE GATEWAY DRUG

People often tell me they either can't find the time to exercise, aren't capable of doing it or don't know where to start.

My advice: walk.

That's right. Walking is the perfect exercise. Why, you ask? Because almost anyone can do it. It's free. You can do it almost anywhere. And best of all: you can work at your own pace.

There's also a hidden dimension to walking that most people don't realize. It is liberating. Especially when you're really heavy like I was for so long and it's all you can do. You are making a statement and taking a stand. You are moving your body. You're not taking it anymore. You are fighting back.

It is no secret that countries and societies where walking is a major mode of transportation have fewer overweight people and lower rates of heart disease, etc.

And yet, people put walking down. The results don't come fast enough. It's not hardcore enough. But these people are wrong.

The secret to a walking regimen is persistence. Once your doctor clears you for walking, you start where you are. If you can only walk 5 minutes before your feet start hurting or your back gives out, then start there. 5 minutes a day, 3 times a week.

Then, gradually, after a few weeks, increase it to 10 minutes. And so on. That is what I did. I started at 5 minutes a day and I now walk 3 miles a day. When it comes to staying in shape and keeping the weight off, more than anything, walking is the secret to my success. There is also an emotional, spiritual well-being side to walking. It's like you are in a march to free yourself from an unhealthy lifestyle. Again, you are taking a stand.

Don't think you have to have an expensive gym membership to "work out" and "do cardio" just to get started losing weight and staying in shape.

You don't. Walk. You heard it here first.

WHEN YOU GET TO THE END, YOU WON!

As of this writing, I have lost nearly 400 pounds. I began at 577 pounds.

In years past when I would lose a bunch of weight, I was never satisfied. The more I lost, the more I wanted to lose. At one point in my life, I got down to 199 pounds and still thought I was "fat." I was just never satisfied.

That was 15 years ago. After I gained all the weight back, I always told myself: if I ever get back there, I'm going to be satisfied with what I've accomplished. I'm always going to keep the proper perspective. I'm going to realize that where I'm at is so much better than where I came from, I'm going to be happy.

I'm pleased to report that I have basically arrived at that point. Sure, I'd like to lose some more weight and I likely will. Maybe I will lose more weight. Maybe I won't. But I have told myself this: I am ecstatic. If I maintain this for a year, I will be overjoyed. The concept that I can walk into any clothing store in America and buy a size medium shirt and a size 36 pants and have both of them be a little too big on me just blows my mind. It's like Christmas morning every day when I wake up.

I always tell people (and myself) that a lifestyle is as much about managing your own expectations as anything else. We want it all....and we want it now. But that isn't how it works, especially if you want it to last. I'm never going to weigh 164 pounds like the government says I should weigh. My body is never going to be perfect. My knees are shot from carrying around all that extra weight for so long. I have a curve in my spine from the years of being heavy. I get neck pain when I sit too long. I now have a tailbone that gives me problems. My dreams of becoming the next great marathon runner have been shattered because my body can't take it.

But you know what? I'm alive. And I'm going to keep living. And I don't weigh 577 pounds anymore.

I have arrived. This is the pot of gold at the end of the rainbow. But I'm not done, I'm just getting started. Life is good, my friends!

FAT SHAMING? ARE YOU KIDDING ME?

Recently, some experts have started calling for social pressure to be placed on heavy people to get them to change their ways. The theory is that heavy people can be "shamed" into losing weight.

This is a stupid idea that won't work, for a few reasons:

News flash...heavy people already know they're heavy. This is one of the biggest myths of the overweight - that we don't know it. We need someone to tell us. We need the condescending thin person to make us aware of just how big we are. No, we don't. From the outside, it may appear like we are oblivious to the fact, but trust me, on the inside...we know.

Social pressure will not cause a heavy person to lose weight. Sorry, it just won't work. Aside from the fact that it is cruel and inhumane, it won't work because there is already plenty of social pressure. More won't help. All social pressure ever did to me was make me eat more to cope with it. It will have the opposite effect. I was always very aware of the people who stared at me in the grocery store, the little kids that would run when they saw me, the people who didn't talk to me because I didn't fit their image of what a person should look like. The pressure to lose weight is enormous. I always knew I weighed over 500 pounds and I hated it. I just couldn't (and sometimes still can't) stop eating.

Heavy people aren't going to lose weight because of social stigma anyway. Not once in my 3 year journey have I thought about losing a single ounce because of what somebody else thought about me. I simply don't care. The only reason I am losing weight is for my health. I don't care about anything else.

Weight discrimination is very real and this would only make it worse. The last acceptable group of people to discriminate against in this country is the overweight. I know it because I have lived it and I will never forget it. The way our society treats those who are heavy is already shameful enough...do we really need to make it worse? Unbelievable.

So what is the solution? It's easy for me to sit here and shoot down somebody's idea without offering my own. The problem is very complex and won't be solved overnight. It starts with the kids. Some ideas:

We must immediately get rid of all the junk food from all schools at all levels. Vending machines, junk food in the cafeteria, soda machines...all of it. The school lunches, if the government is to pay for them with taxpayer money, must be healthy. No more pizza and fries. I'm not saying we have to feed kids tofu and bean sprouts, but we can do much better.

Government subsidies of corn must end immediately. Whether people realize this or not, the US Government makes corn so artificially cheap that it makes junk food very inexpensive to produce.

Back to the kids. Schools need to have physical education twice a day. And not the way they did it when I was a kid. The idiocy of having most of the kids run around the track and climb the rope while the heavy kids sit on the bleachers in shame must not be allowed. Make the kids walk. Almost everyone can walk. That is all you need.

Education. We need a sense of urgency around the garbage that people are feeding their kids. If you want to stigmatize something, do it to the restaurant chains and the food and beverage industry. We should not be telling our kids soda and candy are OK in moderation. The message should be the truth: it's poison garbage that will destroy your health and if you eat enough of it, it will kill you someday. We have to make eating healthy cool. Education, education, education. The older generation is probably lost, but we can make a difference to kids coming up.

Hold parents accountable. I'm not suggesting we take extremely overweight kids away from their parents, but it's worth having a discussion. Facts are facts: kids eat only what they're given. If you let a dog eat itself to death, that would be considered animal cruelty. It's no different with children. Parents must be taught to not reward their children with food.

Shut down the weight loss industry. These con artists and thieves thrive on a $60 billion dollar business built on rip-offs and lies. All they do is steal people's money and rob them of their hope. None of it works long-term. None of it. The only thing that works long-term is eating properly and moving your body. Every one of these companies should be shut down, their executives marched out of their offices in handcuffs and their victims refunded their money.

So that's a start. Shaming the overweight will accomplish absolutely nothing. We are a side effect of the American way of life and what it's become, not the cause of it.

AN OPEN LETTER TO THE WEIGHT LOSS INDUSTRY

I am never sponsoring, accepting advertising from, or promoting any diet pills. Ever. There is no such thing as a "fat burning pill." Green coffee beans are not going to do anything to make you lose weight. Ever. You should all be shut down and arrested for fraud. You are deceiving the public and promoting a quick fix that is a lie. I hate you all. Every time I see or hear an advertisement for a weight loss pill, it is an insult to me and everybody else that has worked so hard to keep weight off.

To the diet food companies: You sell a product that pretends to be something like food, except it isn't. How are people supposed to live on frozen dinners the rest of their lives? They can't. But the dirty little secret is you don't want people to keep the weight off. It's bad for business. The weight loss industry is a multi-billion dollar cartel of companies that siphons billions out of people's wallets while promising them the world and doing nothing.

To the commercial fitness industry: Really? Pizza day at the gym? News flash: most people don't even need the gym. Maybe one day they will figure it out. You sell the lie that you can go to the gym and look like a movie star. The truth is, most people never will. And if everybody that signed up for your gym actually went to it, it would be so crowded you would be run out of business. There are legitimate gyms like the one I go to and I appreciate those. But for most people, if you want to "work out," go for a walk. And then do it again tomorrow.

To the home workout equipment industry: What a sweet scam you're running. You sell people workout equipment that winds up collecting dust and being used to dry laundry. And what exactly does that weight you shake in your hand do? It's not for losing weight, I'll tell you that.

To the restaurant industry: No, I am never coming back. Why? Because your "healthy options" almost never are. Sure, it's only 500 calories...but it's loaded with enough sodium to give a rhinoceros high blood pressure. All you care about is making as much money as possible. There's nothing wrong with that, but you don't care about anyone's health and never will, so stop pretending you do.

To the big, famous diet plans: Most of you are all a scam. Because the truth is the truth: you will lose weight when the total number of calories you are consuming is less than the calories you are burning. Not before. There is no secret plan that will fix it all for you. And no, carbohydrates do not make you fat, you idiots.

I don't believe in conspiracies. But what I do know is that all of these thieves and scoundrels have a horrible track record and I want nothing to do with them. I have not worked for 3 years...and will have to continue to work for the rest of my life....to keep off the nearly 400 pounds I have lost just to sell my soul to these scumbags. Go away...forever.

Pictures

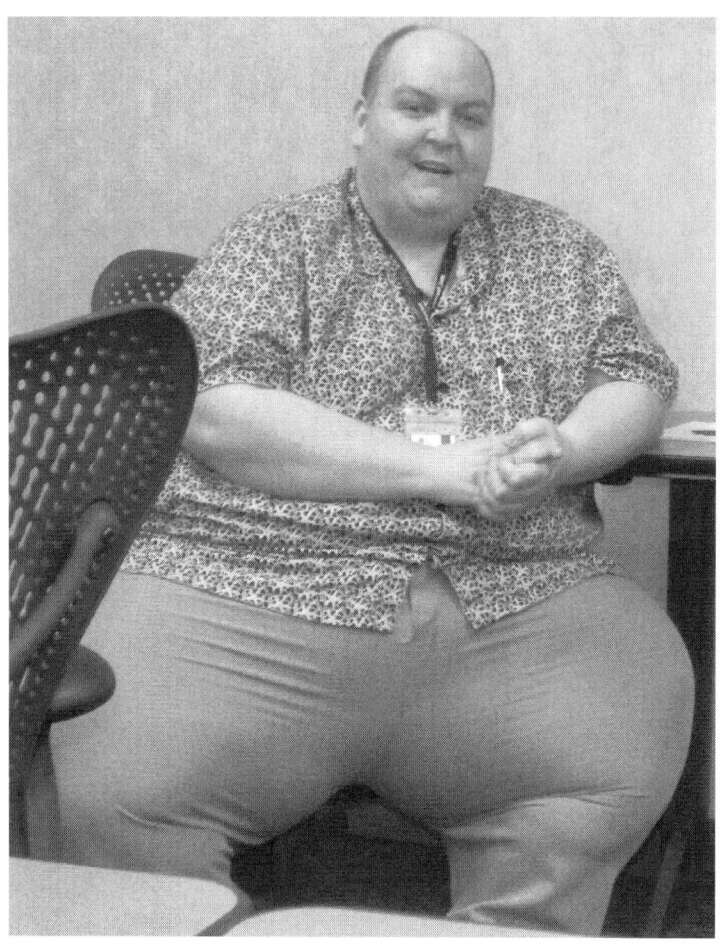

This picture was taken on June 4, 2010, 16 days before I was rushed to the emergency room. I had been suffering from dizzy spells, but didn't know why. I could have dropped dead at any moment. I weighed 577 pounds. (Courtesy of Deborah Hooks)

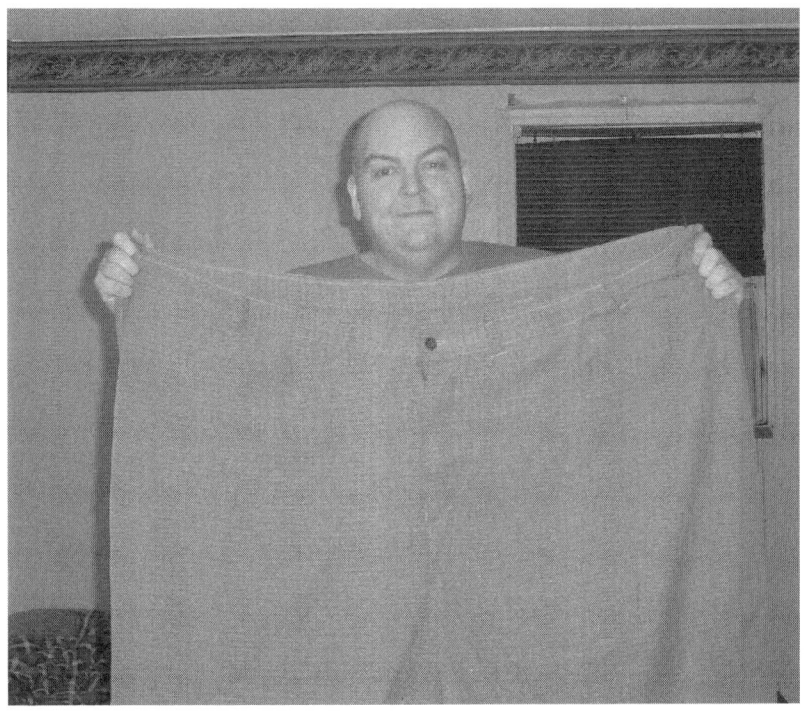

This was taken exactly 6 months later and those are the pants from the first picture. I had already lost over 100 pounds.

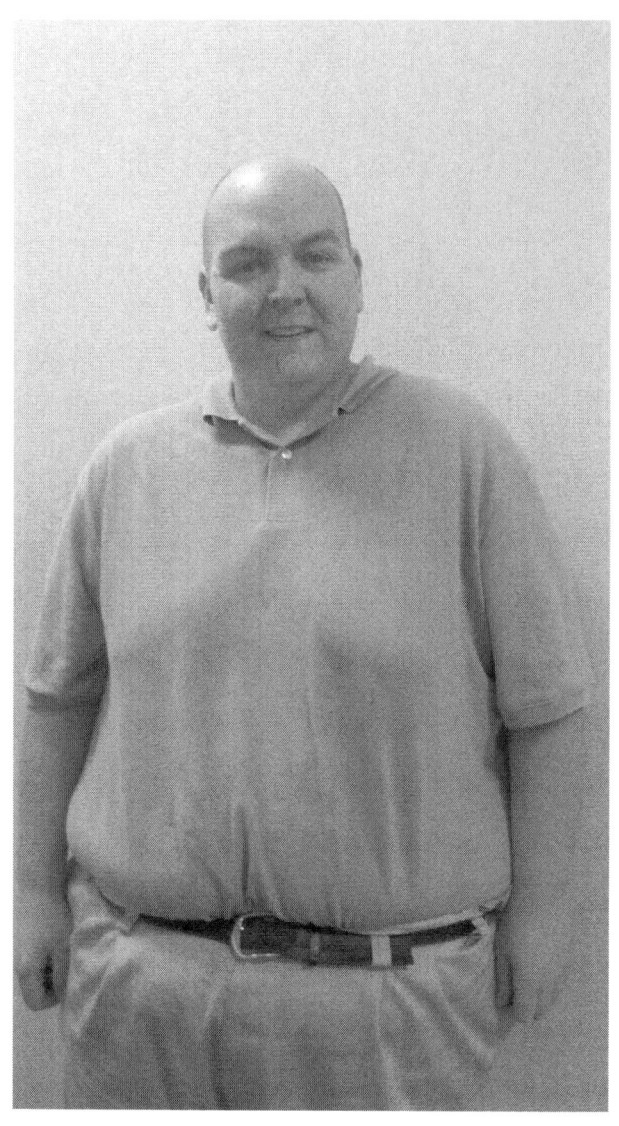

A picture from around the same time. I weighed about 450 pounds. I remember thinking that if this is all the weight I could lose, I was already so much better off than I was. I was wearing clothes from the store!

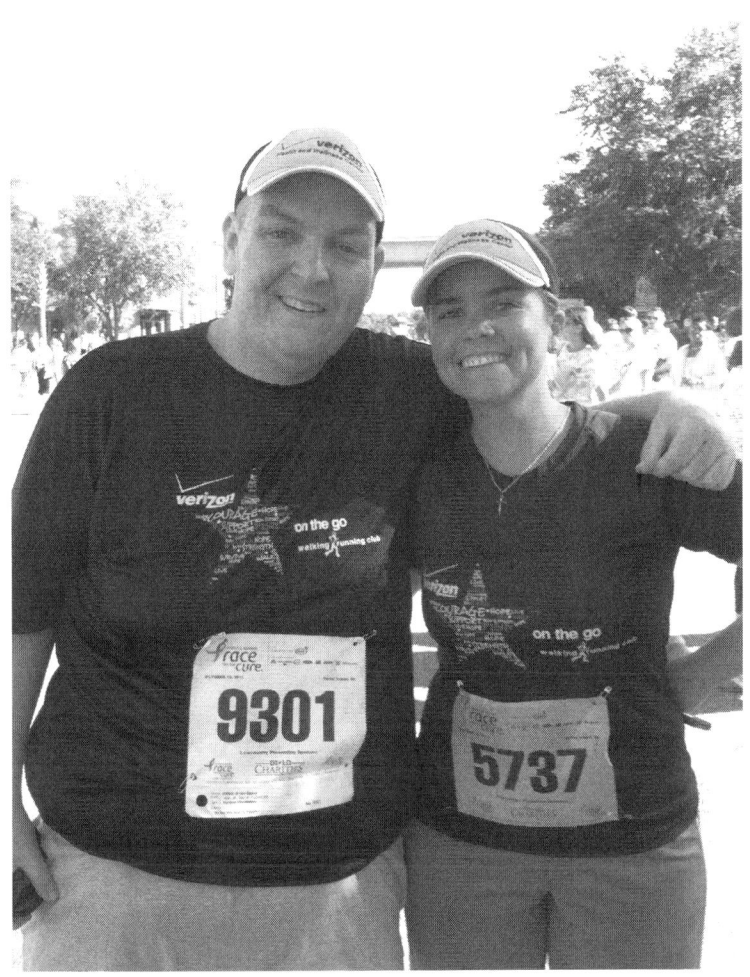

From a 5K race I entered a couple years ago. I walked from the start to the finish. I was living a fantasy. Races were for thin people and I was becoming one. A picture with one of my favorite people, Martha Peake. Martha was my health and wellness coach for the first year of my journey.

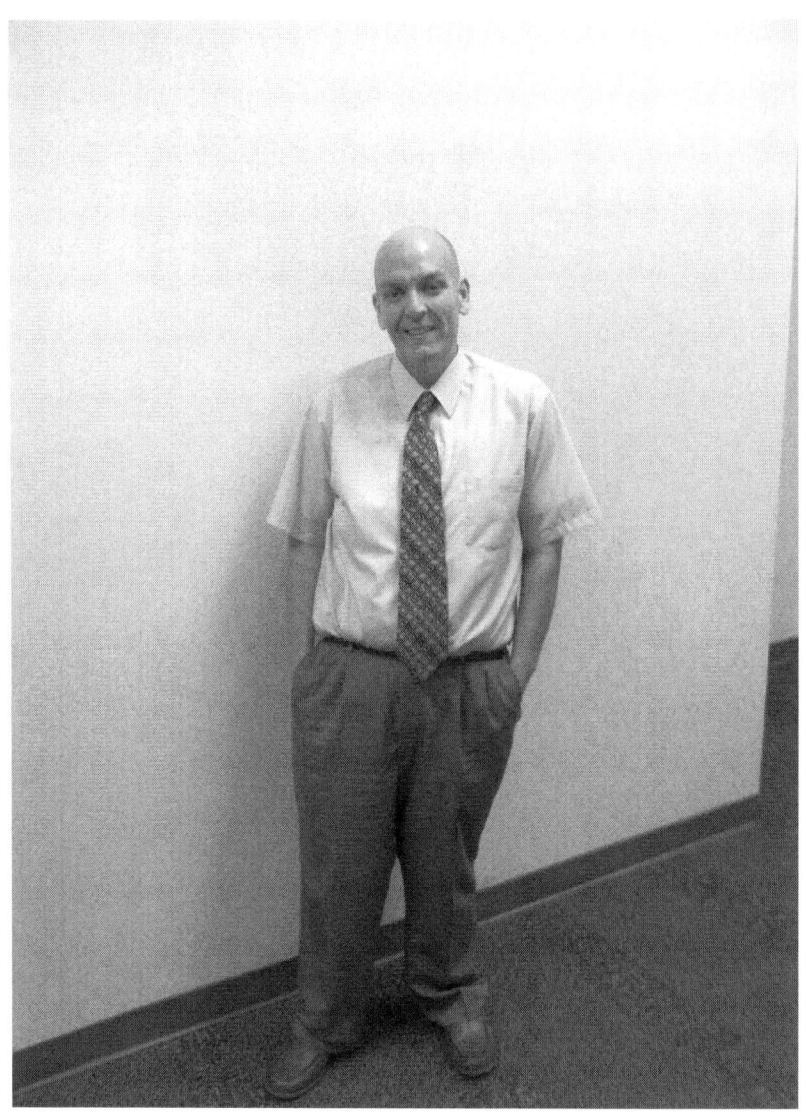

One of my favorite "after" pictures. About 225 pounds. I dressed up for an interview and finally realized I was starting to reach my goal: becoming a normal person.

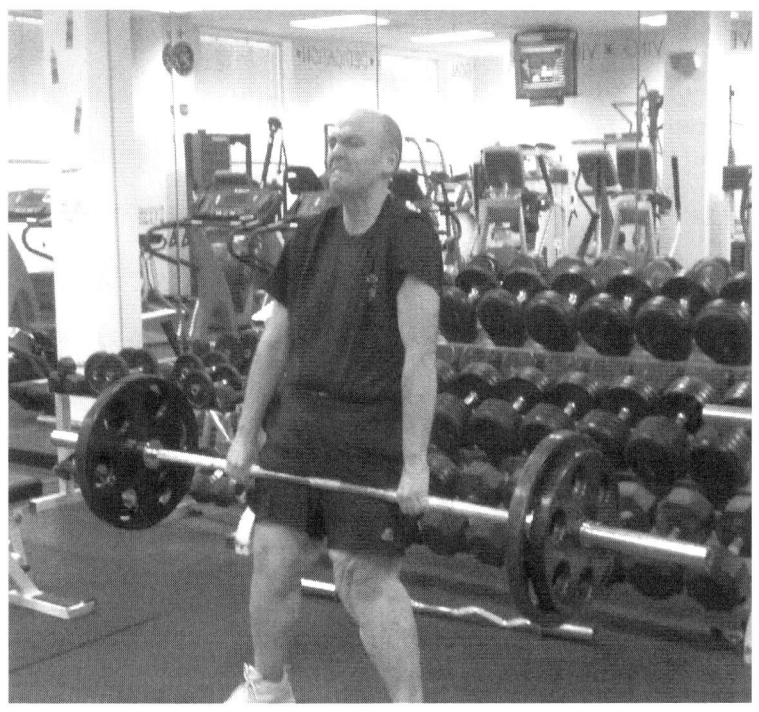

Dead lifting 205 pounds in the gym. I still can't believe that's me, but it is!

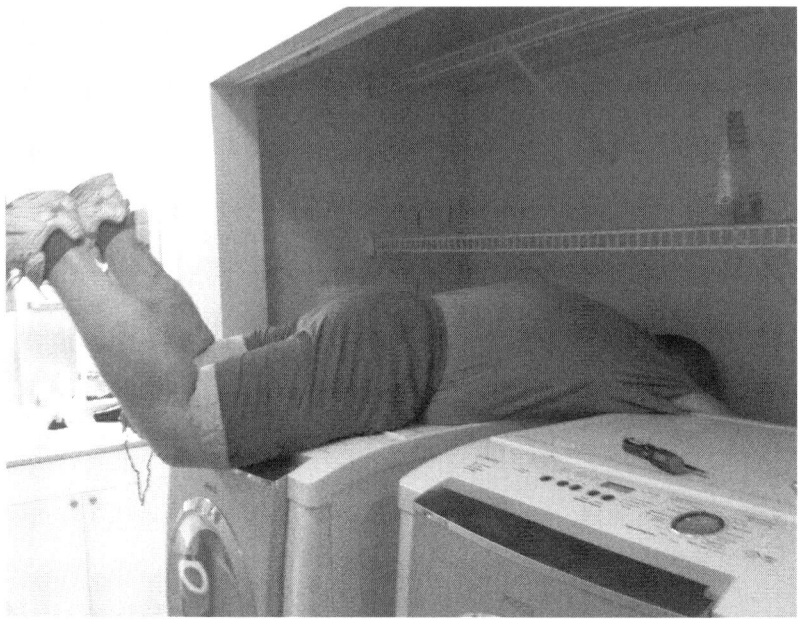

This is when weight loss goes functional. Helping a friend hook up their dryer at their new apartment. I remember thinking I wouldn't have been doing this before!

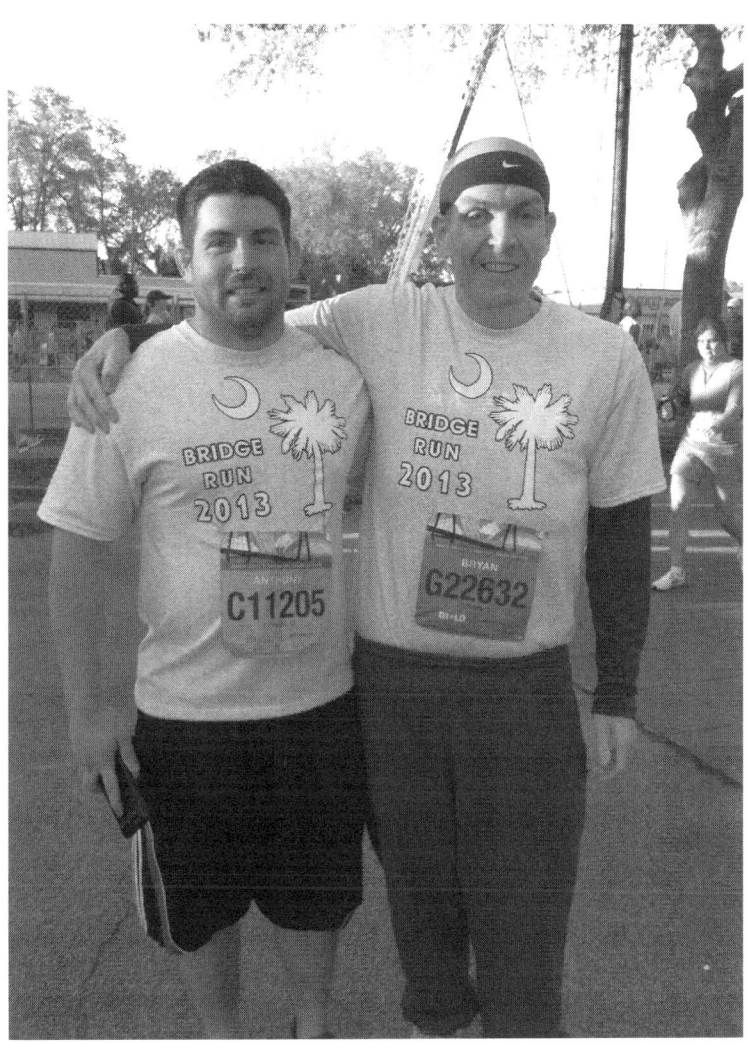

At the 2013 Cooper River Bridge Run, held every year in Charleston, SC. My health and wellness coach for the last 2 years, Tony Smith. This man regularly challenges me to do what I never thought possible.

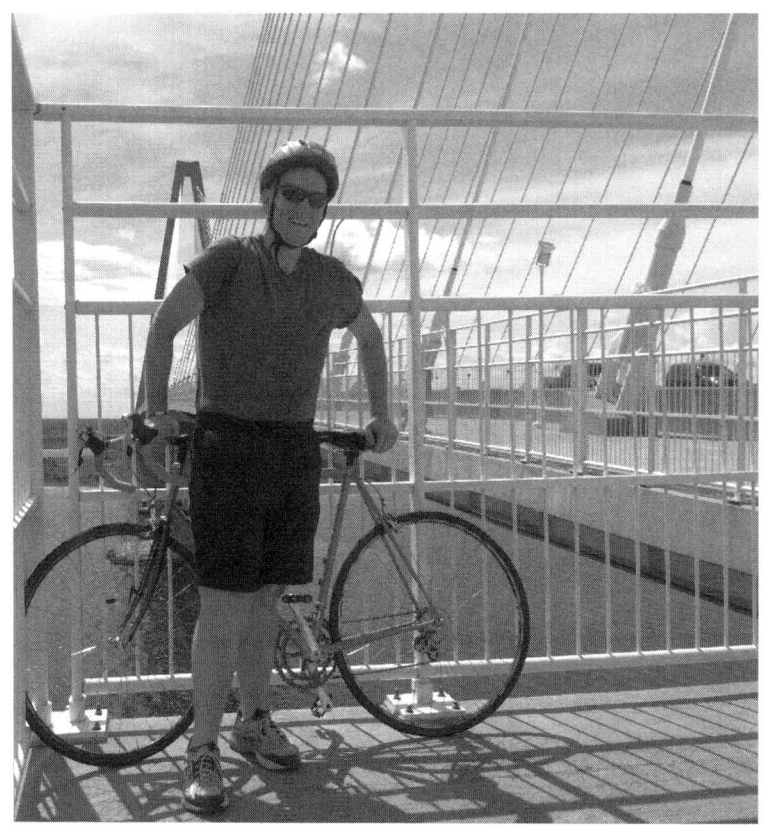

At the top of the Ravenel Bridge in Charleston, SC. I rode 35 miles that day! (Courtesy of Nicholas Honious)

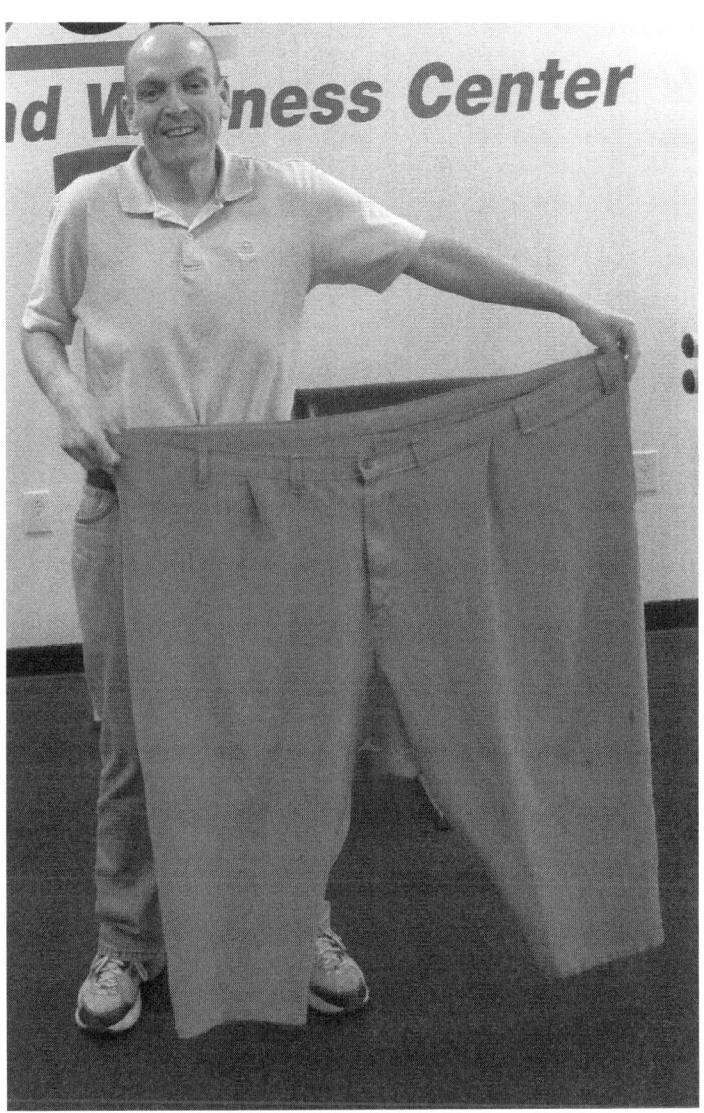

The famous "before" pants. I could fit in one leg now. I still keep them as a reminder of where I came from and where I could end up if I don't keep going.

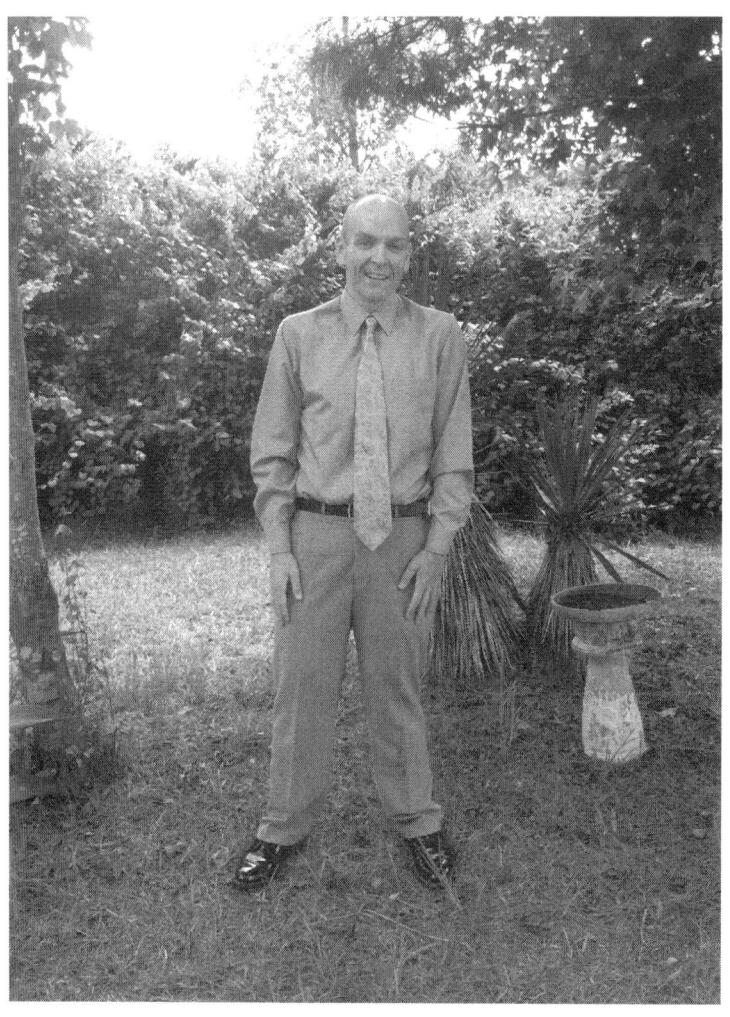

This is the reward. Feeling good, looking healthy and having a few more years added on to the end of my life!

Inspirational... Motivational... Entertaining!

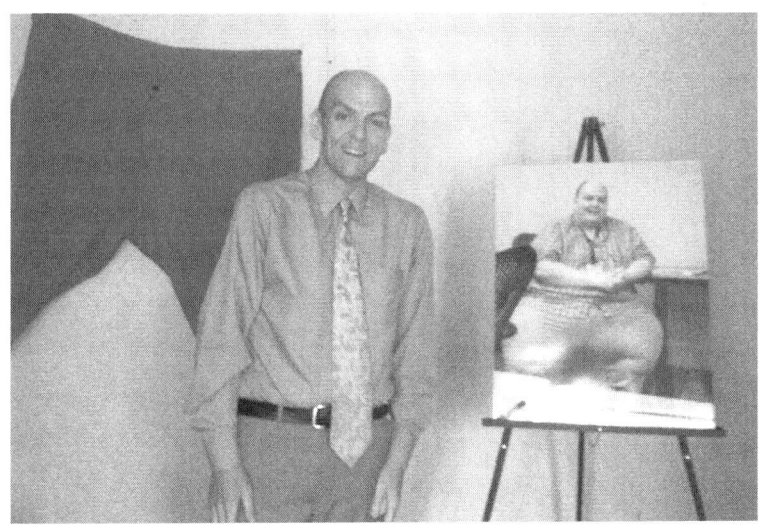

Bryan Ganey is available to speak at your next event. E-mail ganeybooks@gmail.com for more information!

Made in the USA
San Bernardino, CA
15 January 2014